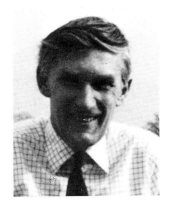

Richa
is Con
Bristo
He is founder of the world famous Frenchay
Stroke Unit, Bristol. He coordinates a close-
knit team of doctors, physiotherapists, occupational and speech therapists devoted to the
research and development of effective methods
of rehabilitation for people who are disabled
after a stroke. In 1976 he helped set up the
Bristol Stroke Support Group to help stroke
patients in his area and in 1983 the Bristol and
Avon Stroke Foundation, to raise funds for
stroke research. In 1978 he assisted with setting
up the Society for Research and Rehabilitation.
Dr Langton Hewer is married with three
children and lives in Bristol.

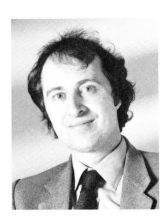

Derick T. Wade, MD, BChir, MRCP has recently
taken up an appointment as Consultant in
Neurological Rehabilitation at Rivermead
Rehabilitation Centre, Oxford. He was
previously Neurology Research Registrar at the
Frenchay Stroke Unit, Bristol, where he
collaborated with Dr Langton Hewer on
developments in rehabilitation techniques for
people recovering from a stroke. Dr Wade is
married with three children.

STROKE
A practical guide towards recovery

Richard Langton Hewer, M.D.

and

Derick T. Wade, M.D.

Foreword by

John R. Derrick, M.D.
Professor of Surgery
Thoracic and Cardiovascular Surgery Division
University of Texas Medical Branch, Galveston

PRENTICE HALL PRESS ● NEW YORK

Published in 1986 by Prentice Hall Press
A Division of Simon & Schuster, Inc.
Gulf + Western Building
One Gulf + Western Plaza
New York, NY 10023

First published in the United Kingdom in 1986 by Martin Dunitz Ltd., London

This book may not be sold outside the United States of America

PRENTICE HALL PRESS is a trademark of Simon & Schuster, Inc.

Library of Congress Cataloging-in-Publication Data
Hewer, R. Langton.
  Stroke: a practical guide towards recovery.

  Includes index.
  1. Cerebrovascular disease—Popular works.
I. Wade, Derick T.   II. Title. [DNLM: 1. Cerebrovascular
Disorders—popular works. WL 355 H598s]
RC388.5.H484   1986   616.8′1   86-8134
ISBN 0-668-06392-0 (pbk.)

Phototypeset in Garamond by Book Ens, Saffron Walden, Essex
Printed by Toppan Printing Company (S) Pte Ltd, Singapore

10 9 8 7 6 5 4 3 2 1

First Prentice Hall Press Edition

CONTENTS

FOREWORD

John R. Derrick, M.D., *Professor of Surgery, Thoracic and Cardiovascular Surgery Division, University of Texas Medical Branch, Galveston*

For the survivors of a stroke, it is the beginning of a long period of frustrating efforts for the victim to learn again to talk, to feed himself, and to return to as normal a life as possible. Left untreated, the emotional scars and the physical handicaps seem formidable. Untreated, the patient often becomes isolated, unable to talk, tolerated but often misunderstood by family members, avoided by friends who are embarrassed in his presence. The isolation breeds frustration, anger, and even hatred which spawns similar emotions among family members. A person who has had a stroke is apt to shut himself up at home and become afraid of the world.

This book is succinctly written for the professional as well as the nonprofessional. It describes the causes and types of stroke, and the psychological impact on the stroke victim, relatives, and friends. The book then suggests the means of overcoming the motor loss and the mental depression of the patients and all of those who take part in his recovery.

The degree to which an individual patient returns to normal will depend upon a number of things. The age of the patient at the time of the onset of the stroke, the severity of the stroke and the size and location of the damaged area. The patient's environment and his attitude are the most important factors in determining what he will be able to do. The goal to achieve is a happy well-adjusted person who can make some contribution to society, however small. The purpose of this book is to do just this.

INTRODUCTION

Stroke is a frightening illness; it can kill, or leave someone severely disabled. Yet some people make a complete recovery. Its course appears unpredictable. Its very suddenness causes distress, both to the victim and to his or her family. Panic and distress are reactions we as doctors see all too often among people who have had a stroke, and their families, and it is because of this that we have written this book, drawing on our experience of working in the stroke unit of a large hospital and our work together on a research project into home care for stroke.

Between March 1981 and December 1983, we saw more than 550 people in their homes after they had had a stroke, many within a few hours or days. We also saw them three weeks later, and again six months later. At each visit we would be asked many questions about strokes by both the person who had the stroke, and the relatives. Many of these people have made remarkable recoveries, others have achieved much despite being left with various kinds of handicap. Mr Plant, a fifty year old man who was left with limited speech and a paralysed right arm, has found an artistic talent and has already had several paintings exhibited. Mrs Jones, aged seventy, was unconscious for a few days, recovered in the hospital from total paralysis and returned home without any noticeable problems.

Using our joint experience with people who have had a stroke, we aim to help you cope better with the many problems and anxieties that can arise. We answer the wide variety of questions that we are often asked by people who have had a stroke, or who are caring for someone with a stroke. Some of the facts we give may seem depressing but this is because we do not intend to hide the truth. We also include real case histories, true except that the names have been changed.

We are going to explain what a stroke is, how it causes the symptoms – such as loss of speech or paralysis – that you experience, and how recovery takes place. We shall give practical advice on how to make the most of your recovery and on how you can cope with any problems that remain. We hope the advice will be of interest to everyone involved, not only those who have had a stroke and their relatives, but also voluntary helpers, social workers, therapists and even doctors. We hope you find it interesting, informative and useful.

Some frequent questions, and where to find the answers

1 WHAT IS A STROKE?

When we say that someone has had a stroke, we are describing what has happened when the blood supply to some part of the brain is suddenly stopped. What we see, in fact, are the outward signs of brain damage that occurs when the blood supply to that part of the brain is cut off. There are three main factors:

1. It is sudden. The effects of a stroke become obvious in seconds, minutes or hours, rather than days or weeks. The person concerned is usually normal beforehand. Within a short time he or she becomes partially or totally paralysed, or develops some other symptoms (see Chapter 4).

2. It involves the brain. Although what you will notice is paralysis of one side of the body, or the loss of some other bodily function such as speech or sight, the damage nevertheless is in the brain. The exact symptoms depend upon the area of brain affected.

3. It is due to a disturbance of the blood supply to the brain. In one or more ways, which are explained later, the blood supply to an area of the brain is cut off. This leads to the death of that bit of the brain. Whatever part of your body that bit of the brain controlled, it can no longer do so; and this is perceived as the symptom.

How vital is the brain's blood supply?
Your brain is completely dependent upon a constant supply of blood. If the blood to any part of your brain is stopped by a blood clot, for instance, for more than four minutes, then that part dies. Most parts of the brain have specialized jobs to perform. If one part dies, its function also stops and you will usually notice that loss. Most parts of the brain rely on single arteries to supply their blood. Each is like a cul-de-sac, with no alternative way in if the entrance is blocked or otherwise damaged. As any of these arteries (or any arteries in your body for that matter) can be damaged, the form that a stroke takes can vary enormously.

An analogy may make this clear. Imagine your brain as a television set. One day, while you are watching television, the sound may suddenly go – the wire to the loud speaker has burned out. You repair it, but two days later the tone changes suddenly – the wire that regulates the tone has burned out. Sometime later you find that you can no longer receive one channel – its wire has overheated and broken. Some damage may cause little change, and if the wire to the headphone socket breaks you may never notice it. If, however, the mains cable becomes severely damaged your set stops working completely. It is dead.

Well, of course, wires do not exist in the brain. But, to continue the analogy, the equivalent to the 'wires' in your brain are the nerve cells, which are responsible for carrying messages from place to place within the brain. If the blood vessels (the arteries and veins) carrying the blood to and from the nerve cells stop carrying blood, the nerve cells die and their function stops. It will help you to gain a better understanding of stroke if we look at the way the nerve cells and their blood vessels work.

How does the brain work?
Your brain, which weighs around 3 pounds (1.36 kg) consists of nerve cells, supporting cells (known as glial cells) cerebrospinal fluid and blood vessels.

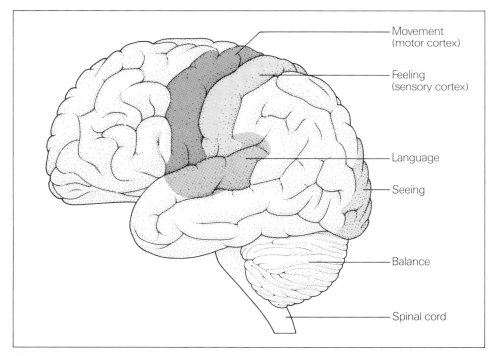

The brain and its functions

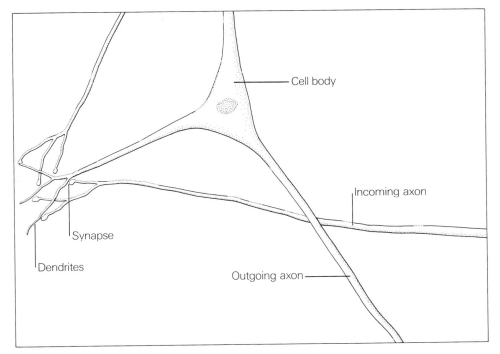

The structure of the nerve cells

It is the nerve cells that are responsible for the brain's functions. Their most important characteristic is that they maintain an electrical potential between their inside and outside. A constant supply of energy is needed just to maintain this potential. This is gained from glucose (sugar) and oxygen, which are brought to the nerve cells by the blood.

Nerve cells (or neurons) are divided into three parts. At their edges, receiving all the incoming messages, are thin, thread-like branches, named dendrites (from the ancient Greek word for branches). The messages are in the form of chemicals that change the electrical potential within the cell. The centre comprises the cell body; this puts together all the incoming information and decides whether or not the cell should fire, and if so at what rate. When a nerve cell does fire, an electrical signal passes along a specialized part of the cell called an axon (from the Greek word axle). The axon is usually longer than the cell and dendrites and delivers the message to some distant point. At the end of the axon, a further chemical message is transmitted to the next cell. This happens at a special junction called a synapse.

Nerve cells usually work as groups, and their axons travel together in bundles containing hundreds of axons (the so-called pathways). The

11

original input comes from our skin and other specialized sense organs, such as the eye, and the final output is to the muscles.

Most of the nervous system is concerned with analysing information and making decisions about it. To do this the nerve cells are clustered into specialized groups, each performing some particular function. For example, one part of the brain simply recognizes that there is a horizontal line in sight. It does not 'know' anything else about the line, but when this is combined with other information, the brain can recognize a dining table, for instance. Similarly, another part of the brain can start with the idea (perhaps a visual image) of a chair and convert the idea into a word, 'chair', which other parts act on so that the word can be spoken.

One of our patients, Mrs Harper, was a seventy-four year old widow who lived alone. One morning she woke up, had her customary bath and went to the kitchen to make herself breakfast. When she picked up her newspaper, she found that she could not read it, though she had remembered to put her glasses on. The next day things were no better, so she decided to telephone her doctor. Again, although she could see the numbers, she was totally unable to understand them. She had to ask a neighbour to come and dial the number for her. She had suffered a stroke affecting a part of the brain specializing in abstracting meaning from letters and numbers, turning them into words and ideas.

Mrs Harper's story illustrates two points. First, a stroke can affect very specialized parts of the brain without causing the more well-known paralysis. Second, it is possible to have a stroke without realizing it. Mrs Harper recovered well.

How is the brain normally kept working?

Blood is the first important tissue needed to maintain normal brain activity. It consists mainly of red blood cells and a liquid called plasma, with two important other components – the white blood cells and platelets. The main functions of the blood are to supply nerves cells with glucose and oxygen, which they need to keep alive, and to carry away waste products. The red blood cells carry the oxygen. The plasma supplies glucose and all other necessary nutrients. White blood cells, whose function is to resist infection, rarely have any function in the brain. Platelets have one important role – they plug any gaps in the blood vessels to prevent plasma or blood cells from escaping. To achieve this, platelets can stick very easily to the inside lining of any blood vessel (artery, capillary, vein). In fact, they are always sticking and the normal inside lining has a system for encouraging platelets to become unstuck.

Another important group of organs maintaining your brain's health are your heart and blood vessels (the cardiovascular system). Blood is kept circulating around your body in various large and small blood vessels by means of the pumping action of the heart.

An efficient supply of blood depends upon an efficient heart. It needs to beat regularly and often enough to keep blood flowing. The blood leaves the heart to enter arteries which are large at first, getting smaller as they reach their destination. Arteries are like balloons, i.e., elastic. When the heart squeezes blood into them, they expand (feel your pulse at the wrist). When the heart relaxes to fill with more blood, the arteries contract, keeping the blood flowing through the capillaries. This fluctuation in pressure inside the arteries is measured when your blood pressure is taken.

Arteries are large blood vessels and cannot supply blood directly to cells. Before nerve cells can use the blood, it must pass through smaller blood vessels (known as arterioles) and enter the tiny capillaries that run throughout your body. It is similar to the difference between highways and streets in the city. Trucks first take the goods along highways (the arteries), then down minor roads (the arterioles) and finally along the streets (the capillaries) to your local shops or stores (the cells). The glucose and oxygen that have travelled in the blood can pass through the capillary walls to the cells. Carbon dioxide and other waste products pass back into the blood. After flowing through the capillaries, the blood enters veins which allow blood to flow back to the heart. The second requirement for an efficient blood supply to the nerve cells is wide enough blood vessels to carry the blood needed.

What can go wrong with the blood supply?

This is considered in more detail later (Chapter 3), but here we will say that it may happen in one of several ways. First, a blood clot may form on the inside of the heart or on the inside of one of the arteries. If such a clot breaks loose, it travels in the blood until it jams in a small artery and blocks it. This type of clot is known as an embolus. Second, the artery may be narrowed by deposits of fat (known as arteriosclerosis or atherosclerosis and usually called 'hardening of the arteries'). If this is severe enough, the blood may suddenly clot on the fat and the artery may block completely with a thrombosis. Third, an artery may burst and the blood pour out into the brain – a haemorrhage. The blood rapidly clots and the artery shrinks, limiting the loss of blood, but also stopping blood passing along the artery. Fourth, the blood may be so thick and sticky that it clots (a thrombosis) as it passes along, blocking off an artery, which may already have been narrowed by hardening of the arteries.

13

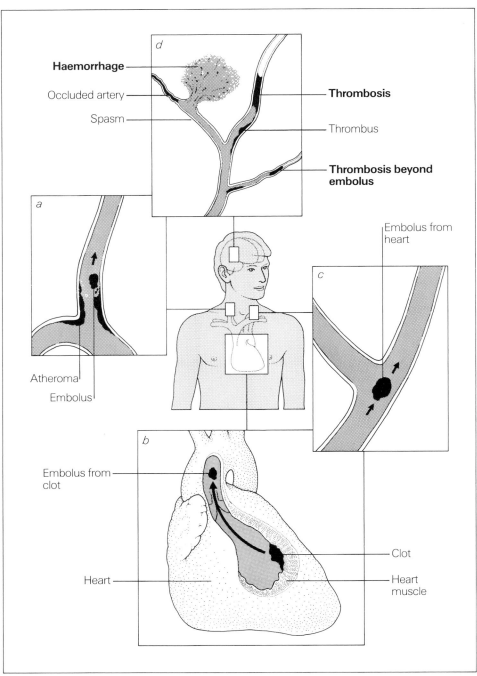

A clot or embolus *a* in an artery narrowed by atheroma, *b* formed inside the heart, *c* travelling in an artery; *d* illustrates the three mechanisms of stroke.

What follows an interruption of the blood supply?

Once the blood supply is cut off, the cells supplied by that artery start to produce more acid, which rapidly damages the cells. At first the cells stop working properly, but remain alive. Within four to eight minutes irreversible damage takes place and the cells inevitably die. So the loss of the blood supply causes the death of all the cells within an area of the brain: this is sometimes referred to as cerebral infarction (brain tissue death). If a reduced supply of blood is available, some cells may stop functioning but survive and recover later, when a better supply is restored.

If the nerve cell's main cell body dies, its dendrites and axons die too. The axons, which may be many centimetres long, depend upon adequate blood supply to their supporting cells all along their length. If the blood supply to any part of the axon is destroyed, then the entire axon from that point onward dies too. Sometimes the nerve cell supplying the axon may die later, although not inevitably. However, the axon does not regrow. Not only are the specialized functions of any nerve cells lost, but the information carried down any axons that cross the affected part of the brain is also disturbed. These disturbances are in fact a stroke.

Some confusions about stroke

Heart attack is one of the diseases that is most often confused with a stroke. A stroke is not the same as a heart attack. The term heart attack may have several meanings, but they all involve some disturbance of the blood supply to the heart muscle. What usually happens then is that some heart muscle dies. It is a similar process to a stroke, but it is the heart and not the brain that is affected. As a heart attack can also happen suddenly, is sometimes fatal, is sometimes referred to as a 'seizure', and sometimes may cause loss of consciousness, it is not surprising that people are confused.

An epileptic seizure can also be mistaken for a stroke. This misunderstanding may arise for several reasons. First, both may be called, loosely, 'seizures'. Second, some people have an epileptic seizure when they have their stroke, or some time afterwards. Third, some people can be left with a temporary paralysis for up to four days after an epileptic seizure (usually any paralysis only lasts an hour or so). The difference between a stroke and epilepsy is important. The main abnormality in epilepsy is an 'electrical' one: the brain suddenly has an uncontrolled, abnormal electrical discharge, but no permanent damage is done. The primary problem with a stroke is in the blood supply, and permanent damage does occur. Although it is not uncommon for a stroke to cause epilepsy, epilepsy does not cause a stroke and is quite different from a stroke.

Other kinds of brain damage should not be confused with a stroke. In particular, neither symptoms following a head injury nor multiple sclerosis (a disease of the nerve tissue) are a stroke. With these diseases, the primary cause of brain damage is not the loss of a good blood supply. The confusion here may arise because sometimes the symptoms are similar. As we mention in Chapter 5, it is sometimes difficult to distinguish between these diseases and a stroke in the early stages.

Mr Harvey, a sixty-four year old retired barman, was admitted to the hospital with severe chest pain. Our investigation showed that he had had a myocardial infarction (heart tissue death) due to thrombosis of one of his coronary arteries. In other words, a piece of his heart muscle died after a clot of blood had blocked an artery supplying blood to part of his heart.

Over the next two days a clot formed on the dead muscle inside his heart. At three in the afternoon he suddenly noticed that he could no longer see the lefthand half of the television set. A clot of blood had broken off inside his heart and lodged in his brain, destroying part of his brain which 'saw' the lefthand side of the television.

Mr Harvey recovered well and returned home a week later.

Mr Harvey had loss of blood supply in two places. The first, in his heart, was due to thrombosis and led to the death of some of his heart muscle. It was not a stroke. The second, in his brain, was caused by an embolus (a piece of blood clot from the heart) and led to a stroke. He did notice his loss immediately but, like Mrs Harper, he had no paralysis. His case also illustrates one point which is discussed in the next chapter: people with any sort of arterial disease have a higher risk of a stroke.

In this chapter we have seen how the normal working of the brain depends upon nerve cell activity, which in turn depends upon a constant supply of blood. A stroke is the outward sign of nervous tissue being lost in the brain, which arises from a loss of blood supply to part of the brain. The wide range of symptoms that can occur, as seen in the case histories, depends on the difference in size and site of the damaged area. In the following chapters we describe the likely reasons for someone having a stroke, and the different sorts of stroke that may occur.

2 WHO IS AT RISK?

Strokes are common. Most of us have a friend or relative who has had a stroke. It is also well known that stroke is, by and large, a disease of the elderly. However, it is not much comfort to you or your family to know that stroke is a common disease among elderly people. What you will want to know is: *Why has it affected me? – or my relative?*

The answer must be that there is not enough yet known to answer that question fully. No one can say why you should have a stroke at a precise time on a precise day. We can only say that because of what was happening in your body you were at risk of having a stroke. We should also point out that the same things were happening in other people's bodies but they didn't have, and may never have strokes. Why this should be is as complicated and as puzzling as why some heavy cigarette smokers get lung cancer while others never do.

How common is stroke?

Every year some 110,000 people in the United Kingdom have a stroke. The approximate figures for other countries are 415,000 in the United States, 50,000 in Canada and 25,000 in Australia. Put another way, a general hospital will serve a population of 250,000 people. In this population 500 will have a stroke each year. These figures are obviously estimates, and are based upon recent research at the University of Oxford, England. Research from the Mayo Clinic in Rochester, USA suggests that the figures are dropping. This may be happening in other Western countries, but there is little evidence at present.

There are other ways of emphasizing how common strokes are. First, they are one of the three most common causes of death (along with cancer and heart disease). Stroke is perhaps the most expensive in terms of hospital treatment. Last, in a population of 250,000 people there will be 1500 people who have survived a stroke. Half of them will have problems such as paralysis or loss of speech.

Who is at high risk?

There are certain so-called risk factors. Among these are diseases such as hardening of the arteries; weaknesses such as abnormal heart valves; or just old age. Someone with a combination of these will be more likely to have a stroke. But the connection is purely statistical. Just as the favourite in a horse race is more likely to win but still may not, so someone with an increased risk of stroke may yet not suffer one. What we do know about possible stroke victims is that only a small proportion of those at high risk actually have a stroke.

It is helpful to remember when we talk about risk factors that their overall importance depends upon their frequency. For example, being hit in the head by a bullet carries a high risk of death but this event is so rare that it is not considered a significant cause of death. In contrast, influenza carries only a low risk of death but it is so common that each year many hundreds of people die from it. So we are talking only about possibilities; simply because you or your relatives have one or more of the risk factors discussed here does not mean that you will inevitably suffer a stroke. The factors can be categorized into five main groups as shown in the table below.

Some important risk factors

1. Those causing arterial damage:
   - Aging
   - Hypertension (high blood pressure)
   - Diabetes

2. Those causing thrombosis (blood clotting):
   - Polycythaemia rubra vera (excessive numbers of red blood cells)

3. Those causing emboli (clots) to form:
   - Heart attacks
   - Abnormal heart valves
   - Irregularity of heartbeat
   - Other heart diseases

4. Those causing haemorrhage:
   - Very high blood pressure
   - Abnormal arteries (diseased, damaged or inherited weakness)

18

- Reduced clotting in blood (leukaemia, anticoagulant treatment)

5. Evidence that arterial disease is already present:

- Heart disease (angina, previous heart attack)
- Previous stroke
- Transient ischaemic attacks (mini strokes – see page 23)
- Poor blood supply to the legs.

As we have already stressed, a stroke is the result of a loss of blood supply to some part of the brain. This is usually due to disease of the arteries themselves. So the first type of risk factor is any disease that causes arterial disease.

Clotting of the blood, or thrombosis (see page 28), is the commonest direct cause of stroke. It is probably the reason for over half of all strokes. Although the thrombosis often occurs on damaged areas of the arteries, any disease that increases the likelihood of blood clotting will also increase the risk of stroke. These diseases form the second group of risk factors.

The next most common direct cause of stroke is a clot breaking off from the heart or the arteries that supply the brain, which lodges further on, blocking the blood supply. Therefore, the third group of risk factors includes any disease that increases the likelihood of such emboli (clots) forming.

Haemorrhage, or bleeding, directly from an artery is the third most common direct cause of stroke, and is the cause of 11 per cent of all strokes. Any disease that increases the risk of haemorrhage belongs to the fourth category. An increased risk of haemorrhage may arise because the blood is abnormal, or because the artery is weak.

Last, there are many diseases that will show that someone already has diseased arteries. Arterial disease usually affects every part of the body, so that damage in one place generally means that all arteries have some damage. These diseases are in the fifth category. Of course, evidence of disease in the cerebral (brain) arteries is particularly important.

The importance of age
Old age is the most important deciding factor. A stroke is rare before the age of fifty, and when it does happen, it is often a complication of some other serious disease such as being born with a heart abnormality. Of course, being rare among younger people does not mean that a stroke is not just as serious as for the elderly. But the point is, half of all

those having a stroke are aged seventy-five or more. Of 1000 people in that group, about twenty will have a stroke over a period of one year against about one person in 10,000 from birth to twenty-five years.

Probably the development of arterial disease with age is the reason for this increase. Few men aged fifty, and few women aged sixty-five, have arteries totally free of atheroma (deposits of fat on the inside of arteries, often acting as a focus for clotting of the blood). As people get older, their arteries are likely to become more diseased with atheroma. This is a common underlying cause of strokes, and so strokes are more common among the elderly.

Mr Collins, one of our patients, had always been an active man. At the age of eighty-eight he still bicycled 1 mile (1.60 km) to his garden plot, where he did all the work. He had had no serious illnesses, did not smoke or drink and was not overweight. One morning he woke and found himself totally unable to move his left arm or leg. He made a little recovery, but ten days later suddenly died from a heart attack.

Mr Collins's case shows that whatever you do, you may still have a stroke simply because you get older. It also shows how people with a stroke usually have other arterial disease, which can cause them to have a heart attack.

Conditions associated with strokes

Detailed research carried out in Oxford, England, shows how often people who have had a stroke have these conditions:

Known high blood pressure	50–60 per cent
Ischaemic heart disease	30 per cent
Transient ischaemic attacks	24 per cent
Other arterial disease	23 per cent
Irregular heartbeat	14 per cent
Diabetes	9 per cent

Ischaemic heart disease is any heart disease caused by disease of the coronary (heart) arteries, particularly angina and myocardial infarction (heart attack). Other arterial disease refers mainly to bad circulation of the legs.

Blood pressure and stroke

High blood pressure (hypertension) is the most treatable of the causes of stroke. Drug treatments and changes in diet, especially reducing the amount of salt you eat, will lower high blood pressure quite fast. Research over many years, mostly from Framingham, USA, has shown that the risk of stroke is directly related to blood pressure. The lower your blood pressure, the less you are at risk. More importantly, it has been shown in the USA by the Veterans Administration Medical Service, and also in recent studies in Australia and Britain, that by reducing your blood pressure you reduce your risk of having a stroke. Reduction of your blood pressure also reduces your risk of developing heart failure. However, treatment does not and cannot abolish all risk; even people with low levels still have some risk of stroke.

Three important facts about high blood pressure

1. It is rarely a specific disease. There is a wide range of blood pressure, just as height varies between people. Various levels have been used to separate people with high blood pressure from those whose blood pressure is 'normal'. Similarly, some people may describe anyone over 5 ft 10 in (1.55 m) as tall, whereas other people may say someone was tall only if he was over 6 ft (1.82 m). In both cases the separation is artificial. We still have to discover at what level your blood pressure has to be before treatment is necessary. The lower the level at which treatment is thought worthwhile, the more people will be taking treatment which may well not be needed. In other words, is it reasonable to ask 5000 people to take treatment to prevent five from having strokes, particularly if fifty suffer side effects from treatment?

2. High blood pressure itself rarely causes symptoms. It certainly does not cause a headache. Therefore, you cannot know whether or not you have high blood pressure unless your blood pressure is measured. A single reading may not always be reliable and so most doctors will check the blood pressure two or three times before recommending treatment. As up to 70 per cent of strokes occur in people with high blood pressure, and as well over half of these people are not being treated at all, it is very important to have your blood pressure checked. If doctors could identify and treat everyone with especially raised blood pressure, we could reduce the number of strokes. You could be saved. Do have your blood pressure checked at least every two to three years.

3. Hypertension is a prolonged high level of blood pressure, not brief periods of raised blood pressure. Most people know that hard mus-

cular straining, such as lifting a heavy weight, excitement, watching television and sexual intercourse can all lead to quite dramatic increases in blood pressure. But this does not increase your risk of having a stroke. It is the overall average of your pressure that is more important. A prolonged small increase in blood pressure damages your arteries; a brief large increase has no effect.

Mrs Jane Jones, when she was fifty-five, was found to have elevated blood pressure when she went into the hospital for a hernia operation. She took treatment for a few months but then stopped. Her husband explained that this was partly because the pills made her feel odd and partly because one day her doctor said, 'Good. Your blood pressure is normal now.' She thought that she need no longer take her pills. Fifteen years later she was seen in our unit, having lost all use of speech due to a stroke. Five years later she died from a second stroke.

Mrs Jones's case illustrates three points. First, most people have their high blood pressure discovered accidentally when being checked for another condition. Second, effective treatment should return the blood pressure to normal, but treatment needs to be continued to keep

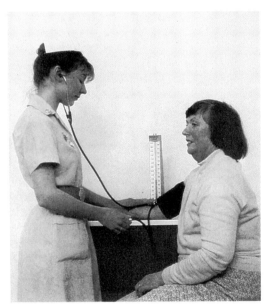

Have your blood pressure checked regularly – it could reduce your risk of having a stroke.

22

it normal. Third, people often have high blood pressure for very many years before it causes any problem.

High blood pressure is usually an indirect cause of a stroke. The longer your elevated blood pressure remains unchecked, the more it damages your arteries, leading at first to fatty deposits (atheroma) and eventually to considerable narrowing of the arteries with a risk of complete blockage. Prolonged high blood pressure not only causes fatty deposits on the inside wall of your arteries, but also may weaken the walls directly. At times little balloon-like swellings, known as aneurysms, can occur. They are similar to the way the inner tube of a tyre may bulge through a hole in the outer tube before bursting. Last, though rarely, excessively high blood pressure may bring on a cerebral haemorrhage. (For more information about this condition and its treatment, see *High Blood Pressure* by Dr Eoin O'Brien and Dr Kevin O'Malley, also in this series.)

Why is heart disease associated with stroke?
Although they are different, heart disease and stroke are often associated with one another. This is not surprising for, as we have already said, all strokes and a lot of heart disease are due to disease of the arteries. As this is usually spread all over the body, one person is likely to have both diseases.

There are other reasons why they are associated. The first is that emboli (clots) floating around in the blood stream may start from the heart. One of the places they can begin is in a damaged area of the heart (such as dead heart muscle after a heart attack, or abnormal heart valves) where clots are more likely to form. Another cause of emboli is irregularity of the heartbeat. It can happen that the upper part of the heart contracts irregularly and does not really beat sufficiently well to empty all the blood. The stagnant blood tends to form clots which may then become emboli. There is another unusual way in which heart disease might cause stroke. Some irregularities of heartbeat can lead to such low blood pressure that blood can no longer flow through already narrowed arteries. A stroke follows.

Transient ischaemic attacks (small strokes)
Transient ischaemic attacks or transient ischaemic episodes (transient = short; ischaemic = without blood) are often caused by disease of the brain's blood supply. Damage to the arteries supplying our brains may take three forms:

1. It may give no symptoms, or signs. This is probably very common, as we know that most of us have some damage to the arteries supplying the brain by the age of sixty.

2. It may occasionally cause temporary loss of the blood supply to part of the brain. This may last anything up to twenty-four hours, during which the person has all the usual symptoms and signs of a stroke, but makes a full recovery before the end of that time. For example, someone might have paralysis of an arm for an hour. Most episodes are short, lasting only between thirty and ninety minutes. They are known as transient ischaemic attacks (TIAs).

We do not know exactly what happens during a transient ischaemic attack, though it is likely that small emboli arise from areas of damage in the arteries in the neck and travel through the brain, breaking up before any permanent damage is done. The exact risk of someone who has had TIAs going on to have a stroke is probably between 10 per cent and 20 per cent over a two-year period. The risk of a heart attack is certainly higher.

3. Most people who have had a stroke have disease of their cerebral arteries. They stand a 10 per cent risk of recurrent stroke each year, and about the same risk of a fatal heart attack. This is discussed in more detail in Chapter 11.

The surprising aspirin   It is likely that simple aspirin can reduce your risk of developing a stroke or heart attack – if you have already had a stroke or transient ischaemic attack. The best amount to take is not certain, but one adult tablet (300 mg) each day seems reasonable. The beneficial effect of aspirin is probably due to its power to thin the blood and so reduce the risk of thrombosis.

From arterial disease to stroke

Aging, high blood pressure and diabetes all increase your risk of a stroke by damaging your arteries. This damage takes the form of a fatty coating lining the inner wall of your arteries, and may lead to stroke in several ways. Very occasionally, the damage may weaken the artery so much that it bursts, leading to a haemorrhage. Sometimes the fatty deposits become so thick that they block the artery completely. More often, the damaged arterial wall acts as a point where blood can clot (thrombosis). This blood clot may then either completely block the artery, or may break off and form an embolus, which blocks the artery further on.

Blood abnormalities and stroke   Normal blood will tend to clot on damaged areas, but if your blood is abnormal in a way that increases the likelihood of clotting, this will obviously increase the risk of a stroke. Luckily, such diseases are rare – one is polycythaemia rubra vera. Anyone with this disease produces too many red blood cells, which makes the blood very viscous, or sticky. If you a: : found to have a disease such as this you will be given treatment to decrease the chances of thrombosis.

Haemorrhage   One important cause of haemorrhage, although not a common one, is when the blood clots less well than usual. This may be the result of many blood disorders, such as leukaemia. It is also possible that drugs to reduce blood clotting can produce a haemorrhage. So any benefit from the drugs needs to be weighed against this slight risk (between 3 and 5 per cent per year).

Diabetes and stroke
Diabetes is one of several other diseases that leads to arterial damage. Recent research from Oxford, England, suggests that 6 to 12 per cent of people who have a stroke have diabetes. However, diabetes is also common among the elderly, so we cannot be sure how far it alone is responsible for strokes. Neither do we know whether good control of diabetes will reduce the risk of a stroke in later life.

Finally, there are a number of factors that you may have thought to be risk factors. They are in fact *not* associated with stroke:

- Smoking: there is no doubt that cigarette smoking does serious damage to arteries, but there does not appear to be a statistical connection with stroke. One explanation may be that those who develop arterial disease from smoking have heart attacks and die before enough damage occurs to their brain arteries.

- Exercise, or the lack of it: taking regular exercise may reduce your risk. There is no evidence that sudden, unaccustomed exercise is likely to bring on a stroke, although violent, sudden exercise might lead to a heart attack.

- Sex and sexual intercourse: are men or women at greater risk of stroke? Men are, or at least were, more at risk of heart attack. This might have been because more men smoked. As far as stroke is concerned, men and women stand an equal risk. Neither does sexual intercourse put men or women at greater risk.

- Diet and obesity: being overweight may marginally increase your risk of having a stroke, but there is no medical evidence showing that what you eat has any effect.

25

- Stress: again, in spite of popular belief, there is no evidence that stress or worry will increase your risk of a stroke.

- Family history: stroke is not an inherited disease, and is so common that chance alone means many families include at least two people who have had a stroke.

In this chapter we have seen how among the important factors which may determine whether you will have a stroke, some, especially age, are unavoidable. Others cannot yet be treated, but one factor which can be controlled effectively is high blood pressure. Unfortunately though, people often do not know that they have high blood pressure. Besides, many people with high blood pressure are reluctant to take drugs now in order to reduce a possible risk ten to twenty years later.

In any case, you should not forget that most people with these diseases do not have a stroke – they are risk factors and not causes. There is an important difference.

3 TYPES OF STROKE

One of the first things you will want to know if you or a close relative has had a stroke is 'How serious is it?' What you would probably like to hear is that the stroke was a mild one, or less serious than most. Even if your doctor were to give you such an answer, it may still not convey a lot of meaning. What is serious, what is mild? Your doctor's answer will depend on the information that can be gained about the stroke and his classification of the disease. As there are many ways of categorizing strokes, we shall describe some of these so that you will be better able to understand your doctor's answer.

You may, of course, be more interested in the practical problems connected with stroke and not with knowing exactly what type of stroke you or your relative has had. In that case you may wish to pass over this chapter and rely on a simple rule of thumb explanation of the seriousness of a stroke: in general, the seriousness or severity of a stroke is judged by the loss experienced. The worse the paralysis, the worse the stroke.

What type of stroke have I had?

The difficulty with this question is that there are many ways of classifying stroke – it depends largely on what is meant by type. Some of the ways of classifying stroke are listed below.

Some ways of identifying strokes

By cause:

- thrombosis
- embolus
- haemorrhage

By effect on brain tissue:

- infarction
- haemorrhage

By artery involved:

- carotid
- vertebrobasilar

By location or size of affected tissue:

- a hemisphere stroke
- a brain-stem stroke
- a lacunar stroke

By duration of symptoms

- under twenty-four hours; a transient ischaemic attack
- under three weeks; a reversible ischaemic neurological deficit
- over three weeks; a completed stroke

By symptoms:

- with paralysis; a hemiplegic stroke
- with speech loss
- many other symptom complexes.

Causes of stroke: thrombosis, embolus and haemorrhage
The meanings of these words were discussed in Chapter 1, so we will mention them only briefly here:

Thrombosis is the name given to a clot of blood that forms within the heart or blood vessels. Such a clot (thrombus) may grow so large that it completely blocks an artery, thereby cutting off the blood supply beyond. Alternatively, a piece of thrombus may break off and become an embolus.

Embolus is the word used to describe any abnormal matter found in the blood stream. The usual type of embolus is a clot of blood, but it could be a globule of fat or even an air bubble. Emboli causing stroke may arise anywhere from the heart and the arteries supplying the brain. In the heart, blood may clot on damaged or scarred heart muscle (for example, after a heart attack), on abnormal heart valves (including artificial valves) and in stagnant blood, which may occur in some conditions. Any person who has any of these conditions has an increased risk of stroke, particularly if the heart rhythm is irregular as this may dislodge clots more easily. Emboli may also arise from the arteries.

The most important disease that used to cause emboli was rheumatic heart disease. This is now rare, but other forms of heart disease, such as aortic stenosis (a narrowing of the main valve of the heart), affecting both the valves and the heart muscle, are now more important. For example, between 2 and 4 per cent of all people suffering a heart attack will have a stroke within a few weeks, and most of these are probably due to emboli.

Haemorrhage – bleeding into the brain from a ruptured (broken) artery – accounts for about 11 per cent of all strokes. As discussed in the last chapter, most small haemorrhages probably arise from areas of weakened small arteries (called arterioles). One particular form of haemorrhage we have not described so far is sub-arachnoid haemorrhage. The sub-arachnoid is a fluid-filled space between two delicate layers of membrane covering the surface of the brain. Bleeding into this space can cause pressure and damage to the surface of the brain. Many people who have had a sub-arachnoid haemorrhage die, some recover without any brain damage, and a few suffer longterm brain damage (stroke).

The difficulty in pinpointing the cause   While we know a lot about what happens in the conditions we have just described, it is much more difficult to define their role in stroke. There may be combinations of one or other causes, for example:

1. Once an embolus has lodged, another thrombosis will occur in the stationary blood.
2. The embolus may lodge where the artery is already narrowed by thrombosis.
3. Haemorrhage may occur both from an artery already weakened by thrombosis, and into brain that initially died after an embolus cut off the blood supply.

Obviously, it is very hard indeed to classify stroke with any accuracy using this system.

Ultimately, the reason for any classification is to provide the best treatment and advice for the future. Unfortunately, with a few exceptions, no specific treatment will help these conditions. A haemorrhage does restrict the use of some treatments, and so needs identifying. Otherwise, knowing what type of stroke you have had will not influence treatment (we discuss treatment in more detail later).

The outlook   People who have had a haemorrhage may be more likely to die immediately. Apart from that, knowledge of the type of stroke will not help your doctor to make a longterm prediction about your recovery – although this may be possible based on other clues and his experience of strokes. So although most people like to know what type of stroke is involved, there is in fact little benefit to be gained from the information.

The effect of a stroke on brain tissue

Cerebral infarction   The word infarct is used to describe dead tissue, particularly when it dies as a result of artery blockage. The term cerebral infarction simply means that some brain tissue has died after its blood supply has been cut off. In other words, a stroke has occurred.

Death of brain tissue may follow either thrombosis or embolism, and is often referred to as thrombo-embolic infarction to cover the uncertainty of the cause. It is mainly used in contrast to haemorrhage, where the primary problem is a ruptured artery.

Haemorrhagic infarction   This means that bleeding into the dead tissue has occurred.

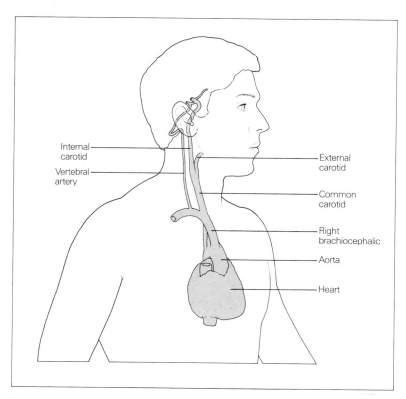

The arteries supplying the brain

Classifying the artery involved – the carotid, vertebral and basilar arteries

Four arteries supply your brain. Two are located in the front and called carotid arteries. The other two, which pass up the back of the neck, are called the vertebral arteries because they pass through your neck vertebrae. In the head these two join to form a single basilar artery, so called because it is at the base of your brain. Further on, the basilar artery splits and joins the two carotid arteries to form a circle from which all other arteries in the brain branch.

As a general rule, we all have the same pattern of arteries in our brains (and bodies). There is little overlap of areas supplied, so that if an artery is blocked, no blood can get through any other way. Therefore, it is often possible to work out which artery is blocked from the area of your brain that is no longer working. Sometimes the deduction is general. Your doctor may know only that the damage is somewhere supplied by the vertebral or basilar arteries. On other occasions, a particular small artery can be blamed.

Knowing which artery is involved would be useful only if it were to help treatment or your doctor's assessment of your recovery; if surgery were useful – which it is not – knowledge of the artery involved would be vital. Otherwise, such information is not of any great value as far as treatment goes.

Naming stroke by location

The brain can be separated into two main parts. The first is the brain stem. This is a small part of the brain (about 10 per cent) which, nevertheless, is vital to life. Not only do all messages to and from the brain pass through this part, but also it contains centres that control our breathing, heart rate and other functions. The second main part of the brain is divided into two halves or hemispheres. They fill the top and front part of your skull. They are the part of the brain usually seen in photographs.

A brain-stem stroke is often fatal, because so many vital functions are dependent upon the brain stem. All brain-stem strokes are due to disruption of the blood supply entering through the base of your brain – the vertebral and basilar arteries. It is an extremely dangerous and delicate area on which to perform an operation to prevent further trouble, and so this is rarely possible.

A hemisphere stroke is one that occurs in the upper 90 per cent of your brain. About 90 per cent of all strokes occur here.

A lacunar stroke refers to a small stroke that can occur deep within your brain, usually causing a loss to a small isolated area, such as

31

paralysis of the hand alone. Other strokes could also be named after the areas of the brain that have been affected.

Duration of symptoms

Transient ischaemic attacks (TIAs) By definition strokes must either lead to death or produce symptoms lasting longer than twenty-four hours. Transient ischaemic attacks last less than twenty-four hours and do not kill. Some people have taken this a step further; they have created another category:

Reversible ischaemic neurological deficits (RINDs) These episodes of weakness, loss of sensation in arms or legs or impaired vision take longer than twenty-four hours to clear, though people get better within three to six weeks.

This kind of classification can be made only if there is a recovery. Unfortunately, doctors cannot tell at the time who will recover within twenty-four hours, who will recover within three to six weeks and who will recover later, if at all.

The most important feature of all three types of stroke – TIAs, RINDs and completed strokes – is that whichever one you have had, you are at considerable risk both of a major stroke, and also of a heart attack (see Chapter 11). The figures for the exact risk for each are unknown, but they are probably similar. Treatment for the prevention of further stroke is the same for all three types (see Chapter 5).

Naming strokes by their symptoms

Yet another way of classifying strokes is by their symptoms. The best known distinction is between hemiplegic and non-hemiplegic stroke.

Acute hemiplegia is the term used when a stroke leaves you with paralysis on one side of your body. A large number of people who have had a stroke (around four-fifths) have some form of paralysis. If paralysis is less than complete, the term hemiparesis us used.

Non-hemiplegic stroke is the term used when there is no paralysis of the arm or leg on one side of the body.

There are also descriptive classifications. For example, some doctors talk of complicated and simple strokes: complicated strokes being strokes which include paralysis and at least one other problem, such as loss of speech.

You may find all these terms confusing. Do not worry too much about them. The important points are to understand how your stroke happened and what you can do to aid recovery. This is what we hope to show in the following chapters.

4 THE SYMPTOMS OF A STROKE

By now you should have an impression of the many ways you can be affected by a stroke. In this chapter we will look at some of the more common symptoms that may arise from stroke. At the same time, what is happening to cause each symptom will be explained. There are, of course, very many symptoms; some are much more common than others, and we will concentrate upon those. First, though, let us look at one or two general points.

What is it like to suffer a stroke?
Neither of us can write from direct personal experience, but there are many books and articles written by those who have suffered and their stories can give a helpful insight both to relatives and sufferers. Anyone interested in these accounts will find some listed at the end of this book.

About 18 to 20 per cent of all strokes happen while the person is asleep. You wake up having already had the stroke, rather than being awoken by it. For those who are awake when the stroke happens, there are two important points to make.

A stroke is not painful
Surprisingly, the brain itself is not supplied with pain receptors, that is, specialized organs that detect tissue damage and give rise to the feeling of pain. For example, brain surgery can be conducted upon fully conscious people (of course, they need small amounts of anaesthetic applied directly to the scalp to stop pain from the scalp and skull). Some people will have a headache or pain around an eye at the time of stroke, but this is relatively rare and not usually very severe. Pain can develop later because of paralysis, or for other reasons, but even this is not very common.

Would you lose consciousness?
Only about 30 per cent of people who are awake at the start of a stroke lose consciousness, with a further 45 per cent experiencing mild confusion or sleepiness. The rest are fully conscious throughout. Usually those losing consciousness are the ones with more severe strokes; they are more likely to die within the first few weeks and less likely to make good recoveries. Like all rules, this one too has notable exceptions. Most people are conscious and free

33

of pain while their stroke develops, and most can recall its start quite well. Hence the descriptions that have been published.

Early symptoms
The commonest early symptons of a stroke are listed below, showing approximately how common each one is. They are placed in three groups – the effects on your mental state, on your physical functions and on your ability to communicate. Many people will have a wide range of symptoms. It is not unusual to lose consciousness at first, then wake with paralysis on one side, slurred speech and difficulty in swallowing, but to be left only with a weakness in one arm. In the rest of this chapter, more details will be given about some of these symptoms. The way they arise and the effects they may have will also be discussed.

Common early symptoms of a stroke

Symptom	Frequency
Effects on mental state:	
● unconsciousness	30–40 per cent
● confusion	45 per cent (of those conscious)
● ignoring one side	uncommon
Physical losses:	
● paralysis of one side	50–80 per cent
● difficulty in swallowing	30 per cent
● alterations to touch and feeling	25 per cent
● disturbance of vision	7 per cent
Effects on communication (if conscious):	
● slurring of speech	35–50 per cent
● loss of language	30 per cent

What causes paralysis?

Paralysis, from a complete loss of any movement to slight weakness, is the best known symptom of a stroke. It is also probably the single most common symptom, affecting about 50 to 80 per cent of stroke victims.

However, to know how muscles are stopped from working, we must first look at how they normally perform their tasks. As a simplification, consider that a movement, for example, picking up this book, starts as an abstract wish, which somehow reaches consciousness. Once action is desired, many parts of the brain become active. The first recordable activity is found in parts of the brain known as the pre-motor cortex and the motor cortex (see the illustration on page 10). From here messages (nerve impulses) travel down through various relay stations and coordinating centres. These have complicated interrelationships that we do not fully understand. Finally, a series of commands passes down the spinal cord to the nerve cells that link directly to the muscles concerned. These commands make sure that each muscle contracts and relaxes at exactly the right moment. They also maintain a suitable background activity in other muscles (known as tone) so that, for example, your arm remains held in the air as you hold the book open. There are over thirty individual muscles in one arm, and each of these has to be coordinated for the simple action of picking up a book, not to mention the need to adjust your posture and balance.

Damage to any part of this long pathway from brain to muscle will disturb muscle control. The places where damage usually occurs are the pre-motor and motor cortex, or the nerve axons as they pass from the cerebral hemispheres into the brain stem. Damage in these areas leads to paralysis – just how much depends on the place and size of the damaged area of brain. If the paralysis is less than total, the more skilled movements, such as holding a pen, are usually the first to be affected and last to return to normal, whereas less skilled movements, such as bending an arm up are more likely to be left intact. Damage to the cerebellum (which is smaller than the cerebrum and lies at the back of the skull) or its associated pathways is less common. When damage does occur there, it tends to disrupt the coordination of the muscles, leading to strong but clumsy movements, so that it is difficult to stand or walk steadily.

Anyone who has paralysis will notice that trying to move at all is a great effort. Any movement is usually slow, weak and clumsy. People tend to describe their affected arm or leg as heavy. As recovery begins and movements do return, strength comes back, but as we have said, fine skilled movements are often almost impossible. For example, the ability to put the pad of your thumb against the end of your little finger is usually the last ability to recover; and many people can carry a shopping bag yet cannot thread a needle.

Reflex actions After a stroke people often notice involuntary movements in their paralysed limbs. One common example is stretching out

35

an arm when you yawn. This is known as an associated movement, and when first noticed it often gives a false hope that some recovery is taking place. But this is purely reflex action, not under voluntary control. It does illustrate though that the brain has some control over the muscles. Similarly, when you concentrate upon straightening your weak leg, it is common for your paralysed arm to bend up. Again, there are obviously connections still intact between the brain and the spinal cord, but they cannot necessarily be used to make planned movements.

What are reflexes? We have many different reflexes, but here the simple stretch reflexes of the muscles are the relevant ones. An important longterm consequence of damage to the motor pathways is that the fine balance of background activity is lost. The best way to show this is by testing your stretch reflexes. If you suddenly stretch your muscle, the stretch is detected in your spinal cord and this causes the nerve cells belonging to that muscle to fire, leading to a contraction which opposes the stretch. This is the reflex. The strength of the reflex (that is, the strength of any opposing contraction) is set by nervous activity arriving from the brain. For example, if you are cold or anxious your reflexes are generally more brisk.

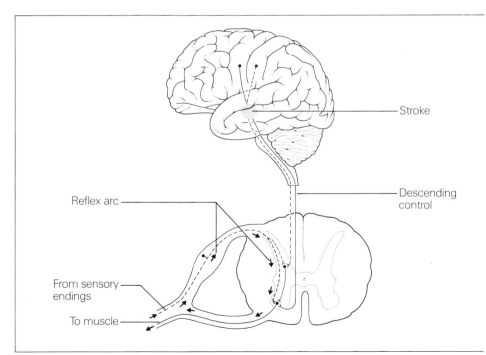

Control of muscle movement and the reflex arc

36

How a stroke affects reflexes   Immediately after a stroke it is usual for your reflexes to be at a less sensitive level. This means that the contraction will be smaller when a muscle is suddenly stretched by the doctor using his tendon hammer. After about one month the opposite occurs and the level of sensitivity usually increases, so that there is a greater contraction when your reflexes are tested. At this stage, it is sometimes difficult to move the paralysed limb because of stiffness, or spasticity (spasticity here means stiffness in the muscles rather than the condition).

You may have jerky and badly controlled muscles if there is damage to the parts of your brain involved in sensation. Normally any movement of your muscles is monitored by those parts of the brain until the action is completed. So there is a feedback of information which is used to correct any change in the original signals given to the muscle. Of course, if the feedback is disturbed, then your muscle control is diminished, leading to clumsy and often weak movements.

Altered feeling

Certain parts of your brain are responsible for 'feeling' various parts of your body (see the diagram on page 10). Normally, sensations arise from receptors in the skin, muscles, joints or other organs. They travel first to the spinal cord, through several relay stations, to the part of your brain known as the primary sensory cortex. This seems to be the first point at which you become aware of the feeling. The various relays on the way are responsible for some analysis of the sensory information, and also for relaying the sensory information on to other systems, such as the muscle control systems. Damage to any part of this pathway may lead to alteration in or loss of sensation. While alterations in feeling are quite common, complete loss of sensation is rare.

From the point of view of the person with a stroke, sensation can be affected in various ways. The commonest, affecting perhaps one quarter of victims, is a realization that touch is in some way different on one side. It is usually the quality of feeling that is lost; silk, for example, no longer feels so fine. This is usually most noticeable in the fingers and hand. It is rare for all feeling to be lost from one side.

Another unusual problem is for you not to know where a limb is without looking for it. Normally you are aware of the position of all your limbs (close your eyes and move your arm – you will know where it has moved before you open your eyes). Even more unusually, some people develop unpleasant sensations so that, for example, clothes seem to cause a burning feeling.

A stroke can and does often affect parts of your brain that are responsible for other specialized analytical or planning actions, such as speech (described in detail in Chapter 9), vision and memory loss.

How is speech disturbed?

In order for you to speak, various processes are necessary (see the diagram on page 82):

1. You have to have some idea or wish to communicate. Disturbance at this stage is called **confusion**; the ideas communicated are all mixed up and illogical.

2. Once the thought has formed, it needs to be encoded: to be turned into concrete words. Disturbance of this encoding process is known as **aphasia**.

3. Once the words have been selected, the actions needed to transmit the words have to be planned; these will depend upon whether you are going to use your voice, or to write the words. Disorders of this detailed planning are known as **apraxia**.

4. To transmit the message a collection of muscles are used. When you speak you are using the chest muscles to breathe out, the larynx (voice box) to make a noise, and the palate, tongue and lips to modulate and control the noise. Disorders of these muscles can lead to **aphonia** (no noise) and **dysarthria** (slurred speech).

How is understanding disturbed?
Understanding requires a similar sequence, only in reverse. The coded thoughts (as words) must be perceived: written words read, spoken ones heard. The messages need to be decoded into ideas, and the ideas understood.

A stroke can affect any of these processes, and may affect more than one at a time. Two particular disturbances are common. First, almost everyone in the early stages has some degree of slurred, or dysarthric, speech, often called blurred speech. This is hardly ever severe enough to make speech unintelligible, but it is noticeable. Second, though less common, there is a more disabling problem when you have difficulty in putting your thoughts into words and in understanding the words you hear. In Chapter 9 we describe how people with language disturbance may often speak quite clearly, but their words carry no meaning.

Physical difficulty with speech
People with slurred speech will notice that their tongue and lips feel clumsy, and will be well aware of this. On the other hand, many people with aphasia do not seem to notice their problem at first. Once they do,

38

they have great difficulty in finding the word they want. They see a pencil, know exactly what it is for and how to use it, yet cannot find the word pencil. You may hear someone use a nonsense word such as 'glomat'; some people will realize that their word is incorrect and try to correct themselves, but others do not realize that they have used the wrong word. It is easy to see why people with aphasia become frustrated.

Less well known effects of stroke

Paralysis and speech disturbance are well known consequences of a stroke; loss or weakening of sight, touch, hearing, taste or smell – and the many others we describe below – are less well known, even by some doctors and other health professionals. The reason for this is probably that there is no obvious external sign. Yet often these hidden problems have major effects upon someone's recovery.

Can vision be affected by stroke?

Yes, it can. Most people blame their disturbed vision on eye problems, but this is not usually the cause. The loss or disturbance of sight is almost always due to the stroke. It is possible for an embolus or thrombosis to occur in one of the arteries supplying the retina (the tissue at the back of the eye that receives the light). When this happens, part or all of the sight from that eye is lost. Yet the loss is often not noticed until you close the other eye.

Normal vision starts at the retina (see the diagram on page 40). Nerves travel from there down the optic nerve, through a relay station to a region situated at the back of the brain (known as the occipital cortex). The brain then analyses the information, building up the image we 'see' in our consciousness. It seems that each part of the brain is responsible for recognizing a particular item. A good example is the ability to recognize faces. A few people have a small stroke that can leave them totally unable to recognize faces. They can tell that the image is a face, rather than any other object, and they can often distinguish two faces as being different: they just cannot identify whose face it is.

One important feature of the visual system is that each half of your brain is responsible for analysing vision from the other side of 'space'. Information received by the right visual cortex comes from objects to the left of your gaze. Objects within your gaze produce two images, one in each eye. These are joined in the occipital cortex. If you have a stroke in the left visual area, you cannot 'see' objects situated to your right. People often think they have a fault with their right eye. In fact, this has to do with the analysis of signals from the left hand retina of both eyes.

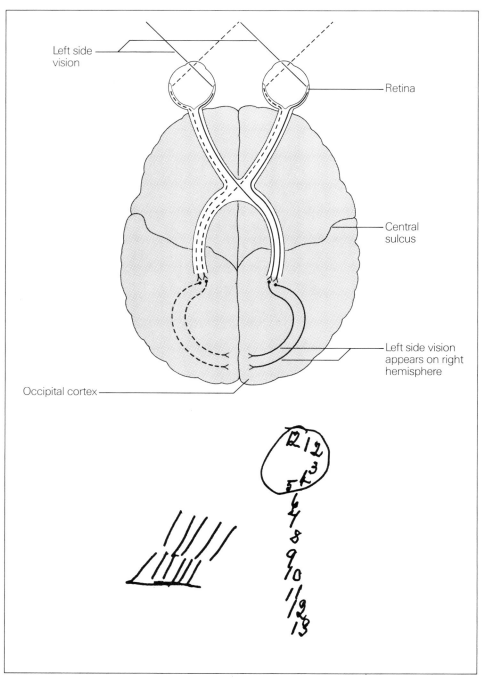

Above, the visual system showing the areas seen by each eye. *Below*, drawing by a woman of eighty-four with half vision or hemianopia. She was asked to draw a clock face but could not complete the lefthand side.

Half vision

When people lose half their vision (hemianopia – without half vision) they can suffer frustrating difficulties in everyday living. They tend to walk into objects on the affected side, simply because they do not know they are there. They hit doorways, knock things off tables, do not see cars coming from the affected side, ignore people sitting or standing on that side. Although hemianopia may affect either side, it is those with loss of vision on the left who are most affected practically. They do not seem to learn to move their head and look to the affected side.

Permanent half vision probably only affects one person in twenty who starts with this problem. For them, driving is impossible and other normal everyday actions become unsafe. Some recent research (from Zihl in Germany), shows that retraining can help. People with hemianopia are often unaware of their visual problem; teaching them to remember it helps avoid the worst dangers.

What other problem can occur?

One extreme example is not being able to recognize the face of a close relative or spouse. A less unusual difficulty is the inability to remember that your body has two halves. This normally affects people with strokes producing a left-sided weakness. They forget or neglect their left side; in extreme cases they may even deny that their left arm is theirs, saying that it belongs to a nurse or someone else. This effect is not restricted to their body. They may not notice objects on their left and even not hear noises coming from their left. Lesser degrees of this difficulty are fairly common, yet may be missed by the people looking after them. If your relative seems to be ignoring the left side, you may think he is not trying hard enough to recover.

Another closely related problem is the inability to organize several movements to carry out a task. For example, dressing may be impossible even without paralysis. Some people cannot make a cup of coffee although they can perform all the individual tasks such as heating the water, taking the lid from the coffee pot and so on. Being unable to plan a succession of body movements is known as apraxia (this was mentioned when we dealt with speech production).

Apraxia is not the same as simple confusion, which is to be expected in the first few days after a stroke. People are not quite sure where they are, what is happening, who is around. Confusion usually clears, but many people are left with more permanent disturbance of their memory and concentration. This, in turn, may lead to difficulties with complicated tasks. While apraxia can affect very simple tasks, such as combing your hair, difficulties with memory or concentration will make newer chores, those that are not so ingrained, hard to perform.

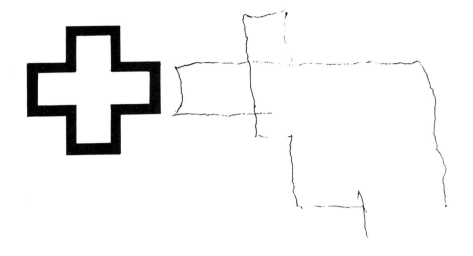

Drawing by a master baker of
seventy with apraxia but no paralysis
following his stroke. He was asked
to copy the cross and had difficulty
forming the shape.

A stroke can cause other disturbances in the way we move, for example, marked clumsiness or tremor, yet without much weakness. We have already touched upon the daily problems produced by disability. In other diseases, such as multiple sclerosis or Parkinson's disease, they are even more common. In later chapters we show ways that these can be minimized, if not overcome.

In this chapter we have tried to give an idea of the way the effects of a stroke happen. We have seen how a stroke often interferes with many systems in the body. It is unusual for only one to be affected. Yet because so much of the brain is involved with movement, paralysis is the most common effect. The brain also has areas with very specific functions. When some of these are lost people may have considerable difficulties without anything being obvious to their families. We cannot emphasize too much that careful assessment by your doctor is needed to discover the extent of any trouble.

5 THE FIRST DAYS: DIAGNOSING AND TREATING A STROKE

Your doctor has four major jobs to carry out if it seems you have had a stroke:

1. To ensure that you are safe; the principal concern is to make sure that an unconscious person does not choke (see page 51)

2. To make a correct diagnosis

3. To decide upon suitable treatment: surgery; drugs; or even no treatment at all

4. To talk to you and your family about the future: after you have had a stroke your doctor's main function should be to teach you and your relatives how to adjust to your altered lifestyle.

To begin with, a stroke leaves the sufferer powerless. Unfortunately, in most cases the doctor is also powerless to influence what has happened to the brain. This is the most important fact to realize about the doctor's role. Television programmes tend to show dramatic operations, and sometimes other treatments. The fact is that for most cases nothing has yet been proved to alter either the amount of damage to the brain or to the process of recovery. This is not to say that no one should have any treatment; a few people may benefit from particular treatments (see page 47). But you should not be surprised if you are not given any – it certainly doesn't mean you are being neglected.

Diagnosis

The diagnosis of a stroke is usually easy, and the people concerned or their relatives often make it themselves. But there is doubt in about 5 per cent of cases. These people certainly need to see a specialist and this means going to the hospital if you have not already been seen by a consultant. There a neurologist (a doctor specializing in diseases of the nervous system, which, of course, includes the brain) is likely to examine the patient. In many hospitals special investigations, in the form of various tests, are considered highly important.

43

There are, of course, several diseases that appear so similar that they can be mistaken for a stroke. Unconsciousness can be due not only to a stroke but also to such problems as an overdose of drugs, diabetes or a head injury. If someone is conscious, it is easier to know whether the attack was a stroke, but there are other possible diagnoses. Some of these are:

- Epilepsy, especially if there is weakness after the attack
- Migraine
- Multiple sclerosis
- Parkinson's disease
- Cerebral tumour.

Of these, the most important condition to identify as distinct from a stroke is the presence of a tumour. About one-third of cerebral tumours can be cured by surgery. This is not a condition you can discover. It will be up to your doctor to give you the right tests.

Tests

The first reason for testing you is to establish whether or not you have had a stroke. The second is to gain more detailed information about the stroke. When considering the need for tests, your doctor will bear in mind three important facts:

1. No test can prove that a stroke has or has not taken place

2. Some tests carry risk, although it is usually very small

3. Tests are useful only if they lead to a change in treatment.

The most common test is a computerized axial tomogram (often referred to as a CAT scan). The machine takes x-ray 'slices' of the brain, showing any abnormal areas. As about one person in five with a stroke has no particular abnormality showing on their scan, a CAT scan cannot always prove that someone has had a stroke. What the scan can do more effectively is identify brain tumours that may initially have been diagnosed as a stroke. Tumours are usually obvious on the scan, although unfortunately not in every case.

The other use of the CAT scan is to detect a haemorrhage. This it can do with reasonable certainty. It will be needed if treatment with drugs that may increase the risk of bleeding (see page 48) is being considered.

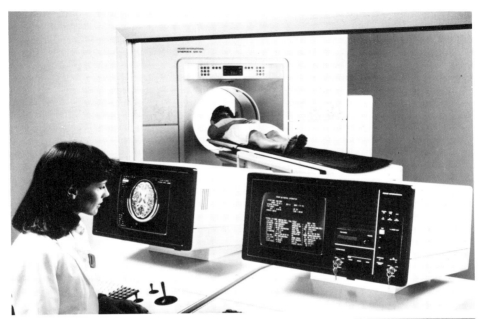

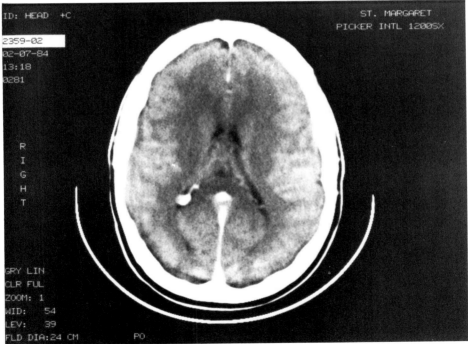

Above, a CAT scanner in operation. *Below*, a CAT scan gives a very clear picture of all the areas of the brain.

A CAT scan, then, has two specific uses: it can prove someone has a tumour, or other obvious abnormality, causing an apparent stroke. In other words, it can disprove stroke. Second, it can show whether there has been any haemorrhage.

Tests have two further purposes. First, they may cast light on some underlying cause. For example, most people admitted to the hospital will have an electrocardiogram (ECG). This test may show an irregularity of the heartbeat, as well as evidence of a recent or old heart attack (myocardial infarction). The second purpose is to detect a possible complication of the stroke. For example, it is quite common for people to develop a raised level of glucose (sugar) in their blood after a stroke.

We were recently asked to see Mr Eliot, a widower living alone, who was found in bed one morning unable to speak and with paralysis on his right side. His doctor had last seen Mr Eliot two months earlier because of a mild headache. He had always been well. The doctor assumed that Mr Eliot had suffered a stroke. With the help of therapists from our unit, he was at first treated at home. He did not recover as expected, which led to some doubt about the diagnosis. After a few days, his son contacted us to say that Mr Eliot was having increasingly bad headaches, and had had progressive right-sided

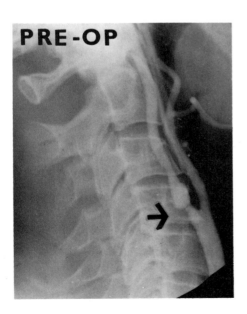 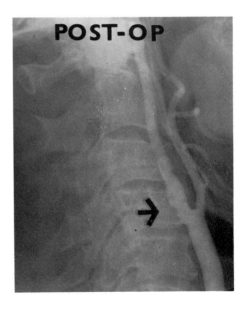

Arteriograms, *left*, showing a carotid artery (indicated by the arrow) narrowed by atheroma and, *right*, after it has been operated upon.

weakness since he had last been seen by the family doctor. This confirmed our doubts. A CAT brain scan was immediately arranged. A benign tumour was revealed and was removed successfully. About two months later, Mr Eliot returned home.

Mr Eliot's story illustrates the importance of understanding the signals of an apparent stroke. It was assumed that his problem had come on suddenly, but in fact it had begun very slowly, which made a stroke unlikely. It shows how another condition should be suspected if recovery does not proceed as expected; and it also illustrates the most useful aspect of tests – in this case we discovered a tumour. The delay of a few days caused Mr Eliot no harm.

Seeing inside your arteries

A common test designed to look at the arteries supplying your brain is arteriography. A needle is either placed straight into the carotid artery in your neck, or a very long one is pushed there from an artery in your groin. Once in place, a fluid (often referred to, incorrectly, as a dye) is injected to outline the inside of your arteries on an x-ray. In this way areas of fatty deposits on the inside of your arteries can be found. However, your doctor will weigh up very carefully any possible benefits to be gained from this test as there is a risk from this procedure, sometimes of a further stroke.

Most people admitted to the hospital after a stroke will have some tests. How many you have will reflect the extent of the symptoms, and the facilities available. In our experience, few people need the more complicated tests. Indeed, we have seen many people who were never admitted to the hospital and needed only simple blood tests. You should not be surprised if only a few tests are carried out, nor feel that tests are needed to prove the diagnosis. Each one carries some risk of an unwanted problem or complication developing. The most important factors are the skill and expertise of your doctor.

Treatment

Diagnosis naturally leads on to a consideration of treatment. It is generally accepted that if your brain is deprived of blood it dies in four minutes, and cannot be revived. We now believe that after a stroke it may be a few hours before all the brain tissue dies. Even given this amount of time the opportunity to stop much of the damage caused by a stroke is limited. Nevertheless, treatments, usually drugs, are given, often many hours or days after the stroke has happened. Sometimes these treatments are to prevent further loss of blood supply which would cause further damage. Sometimes they are given to try to rescue

47

brain tissue that is only just alive, around the edge of the dead brain. Other drugs are given in the hope of recovery.

Anti-clotting drugs   One group of drugs is the anticoagulants, so named because they reduce the likelihood of the blood clotting. Some commonly used ones are heparin, which is injected straight into your veins, and warfarin (rat poison), which you take by mouth. Anticoagulant drugs may be used:

1. As soon as possible, to halt further progress of the stroke in the first few hours or days, particularly if the patient seems to be getting worse or fluctuating

2. Later, to try to prevent further strokes or heart attacks.

Some doctors do not use this form of treatment, while it is quite commonly used by others. There are risks involved in using anticoagulant drugs. The most important is that they may cause serious haemorrhage, and so cause a stroke to take place or get worse. Bleeding may occur elsewhere. The benefits of these drugs have not yet been proven satisfactorily.

Of the many other treatments that may be used, one is intravenous dextran, a chemical that reduces the likelihood of blood clotting and may also improve blood flow. However, it does not help people who've had a stroke to recover, it only reduces the chances of a further one. Steroids (for example, prednisolone) have been tried for the same reason, but again do not have any immediate effect on stroke sufferers.

It is hard for a doctor to tell someone suffering from a stroke – or his or her relatives – that recovery will be natural and requires no drug treatment. Often, pressure to have some kind of treatment is very strong. If a drug is given to someone making a natural recovery, the drug will probably take the credit and then other people feel they should receive the same treatment.

Revival of an old treatment?   One treatment recently introduced goes back centuries – bleeding. The theory is that by diluting the blood it can flow more easily into deprived areas. One study in Sweden showed some benefit from combining bleeding with giving the drug dextran. If this is confirmed, it will be the first effective treatment to improve recovery. It also seems relatively simple and safe.

48

Surgery

Very occasionally it is worthwhile removing a haemorrhage from the brain. However, most haemorrhages are reabsorbed naturally, and surgery helps only when the blood, leaking into a confined area, is pressing on vital areas of the brain stem. Attempts to improve the blood supply immediately after the stroke do not help. In the long term, it is possible that removal of atheroma (see Chapter 2) from the carotid artery might reduce the risk of another stroke. But the operation has to be undertaken with care because it may actually bring on a stroke.

Clearly, much more research is needed to discover safe, effective and simple treatments. Over the years many drugs have been suggested that, on paper at least, seemed to offer some hope. Once tested scientifically, most have been found ineffective. It should be stressed that research is lengthy and expensive. Many hundreds of people need to be studied just to discover if one treatment is effective.

What can your doctor do?

As we have already stressed, your doctor must ensure that the diagnosis is correct. Checking that you recover as expected, with treatment if necessary, will confirm this.

The doctor's second vital task is to prevent complications, if possible, and to diagnose and treat any that may arise. Complications are medical problems that are not recognized as an inevitable part of the stroke itself. For example, paralysis is part of stroke, whereas bedsores are not.

Some complications

After a stroke, people may develop complications of three types:

Due to immobility:
- chest infection
- bedsores
- constipation
- blood clots in the legs

Due to paralysis:
- pain in the shoulder
- joint deformity
- falls

Due to brain damage:
- epilepsy
- pain.

The first group result from your being unable to move. They include bedsores, which can usually be avoided by regular turning and massaging of paralysed limbs, and constipation, which can be helped by a high-fibre diet and drinking a lot of fluid – water, fruit juice or soup. Chest infection, such as bronchopneumonia, is another of these complications which should be avoided. Your doctor should make sure that you receive a high standard of nursing.

One common complication likely to be caused by immobility is the development of blood clots in the veins of the legs. This is known as deep venous thrombosis. In our experience it causes few problems, but very occasionally can result in death if one of the clots breaks away from the leg and lodges in the main arteries in the lungs, blocking most of the blood flow. This is known as a pulmonary embolus. As yet there is no effective, safe method of avoiding the few unexpected deaths that arise from it.

The second group of complications also follows on from paralysis, but these are confined to a particular part of your body. Some people develop a pain in the shoulder of the affected arm. Why they do so we do not know, neither have we found a reliable treatment, other than simple pain-killers. However, it seems likely that you will reduce the chance of someone developing a painful shoulder by not pulling on the paralysed arm (see Chapter 8).

With modern nursing practices and physiotherapy, only a few people who have paralysed limbs develop deformities of the joints. These are called contractures, as the joint is contracted and cannot be fully bent or stretched. Any paralysed limb should be moved carefully, through a full range of movements at least twice each day to prevent contractures.

Falls are reduced by providing help for any difficult movement such as getting out of bed or moving from the bed to a chair and back (see page 72).

Finally, some people develop epilepsy after their stroke. This can be treated with drugs if necessary. Occasionally, someone will develop an unpleasant burning pain. This is rare and the treatment is by powerful drugs.

Your doctor will want to talk to you and your family, to explain the diagnosis, what is being done or not done and why – or why not – and to give some idea of what the future holds. These aspects will be covered in the next two chapters.

6 COPING WITH THE FIRST FEW HOURS

Most strokes happen at home; yet few of us are taught what to do. This chapter should help any reader cope well with most sorts of stroke. Of course, the wide variety of symptoms that may arise make it impossible to be specific about every possible combination. Nevertheless, certain general principles will guide you safely through 99 per cent of cases. In this chapter we describe the course of a stroke over the first few hours, and the prospect of the first few weeks.

Mrs Brown woke one morning to find her husband paralysed on his left side. When he tried to speak, his speech was slurred and difficult to understand. On trying to sit up, he fell to the left. He said he did not feel ill, and she was not to worry. Mrs Brown insisted on calling for an ambulance against her husband's wishes. He was taken to the hospital.

Should you always call an ambulance if someone has a stroke? No. As we saw in the last chapter, there is currently no immediate medical or surgical treatment that is necessary, and so there is no need for everyone who has a stroke to be rushed to the hospital. There are, though, certain circumstances when an ambulance should be called:

1. If someone is unconscious and you cannot prevent an attack of choking.
2. If someone has an epileptic fit lasting longer than two minutes.

You should be prepared for someone who loses consciousness during a stroke to die; nevertheless, this is not inevitable. What is important is that you should not allow anyone who has lost consciousness simply to choke to death. Anyone unconscious from any cause should be turned on to his or her side (see the illustration on page 52). This avoids the risk of inhaling vomit into the lungs. It also makes breathing easier as the tongue will not fall back into the mouth. If you can maintain the position, immediate admission to the hospital is not essential. You have time to call for your doctor and seek advice. However, if you cannot prevent the person from choking, you must call for immediate help.

51

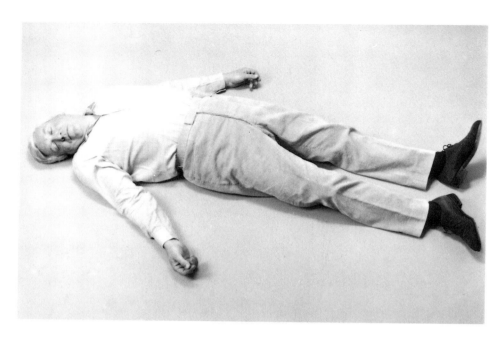

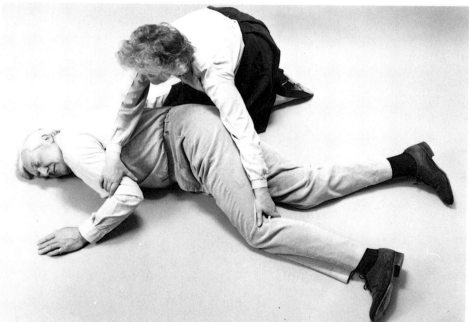

Never leave someone who has collapsed lying on his back as this could lead to choking. Turn him on his side, making sure the airways are clear and with the free leg and arm resting on the ground to prevent his rolling on to his back again.

About 5 per cent of people have a convulsion at the beginning of their stroke. This will probably be brief and it is usually followed by a period of unconsciousness (coma) lasting from between five and sixty minutes. Prolonged convulsions are dangerous. Although most stop before the doctor arrives, no one can be sure when or if a fit will stop. Again, if you see someone having a fit you should lay him down in a clear space where he cannot injure himself. Do not put anything in his mouth – your fingers will be bitten or his teeth will be broken on any object like a spoon. Stay with him, getting him on his side if possible, especially if he vomits. Get someone else to call an ambulance if the fit lasts over two minutes, that is, as long as it takes to ensure the person is safe.

In almost all other circumstances where you suspect a stroke, the wisest course is to call a doctor. The delay before the doctor arrives may well be an advantage. If your companion has only fainted, or had a transient ischaemic attack (see Chapter 2), the rapid recovery before the doctor arrives will make this obvious, and everyone involved will also have at least a little time to consider how they wish to manage the problem.

Should you move someone just after a stroke?   Yes, provided you take care. Of course, if the stroke happened during sleep, it is not likely that you will need to move your relative from bed. Anywhere else, once you have decided that this is not a case for calling an ambulance immediately, you should move the person to a safe and comfortable place. Doing this is perfectly safe, not only for people who have had a stroke but in almost any similar emergency.

The main concerns are practical. Where is the best place? Clearly someone who collapses outside on the street would be much safer indoors. Inside, the best place is usually the living room or bedroom, where there is space and somewhere for the person to lie down. Lying on a bed or sofa is more comfortable, and more manageable for you, than the floor.

Moving will do no harm, but the way you go about it may. You have to ask yourself, 'Can I move my relative to the ideal place for me to cope? Who can help me? Can we do it without causing harm?' It is, of course, always best to have as much help as possible. You must be able to make the move without letting the person fall or be dropped. Neither should you in any circumstances pull on, or allow to drop, any paralysed arm or leg. If your relative is unconscious, be sure breathing is not impeded. Still, many people are not badly immobilized and you may find you need only a little assistance.

To recap, if you are confronted by someone who seems to have had a stroke, do not panic. You are unlikely to do any harm provided you remember to protect the breathing. Whether you need to call an ambulance will depend entirely upon the severity of the attack. But as long as you have enough help, you should move the person to the most convenient place as soon as possible.

Hospital admission

The delay between your calling the doctor and his or her arrival may prevent an unnecessary hospital admission. Of course, in many countries just about everyone with a suspected stroke is admitted to the hospital.

We certainly do not agree that this is necessary for everyone. As we showed in the last chapter, many people do not need the tests or treatments that are provided in a modern hospital. We believe that everyone who needs special tests, and those people who have frequent epileptic convulsions, should always be admitted. Otherwise, it is a matter of looking at your home circumstances. If the right nursing care can be given at home, this is the best place for a lot of people. Families too are often happier to have their relative at home.

What changes may occur on the first day after a stroke?

Most strokes do their worst damage within the first twenty-four hours, although in up to 5 per cent of people, the damage will continue and increase for as long as one week. Rarely is the onset of a stroke instantaneous, but in about half of all cases, the full extent of the stroke will be reached in six hours. On the other hand, many people will show improvement within the first twenty-four hours. Indeed, as we mentioned earlier, some people will recover completely within twenty-four hours in which case, theirs will have been a transient ischaemic attack, not a stroke. A few will show rapid fluctuations, improving and getting worse, over the first twenty-four to forty-eight hours.

What are the chances of death?

This distressing question has to be faced. One-third of people who have an acute stroke will die within the first three weeks, usually from their stroke. Most of them will have suffered some loss of consciousness within the first day, have a severe degree of paralysis and will be unable to look towards their paralysed side. Another bad sign is incontinence. We have found that people who are incontinent after their stroke are more likely to die.

Although these four conditions should prepare you for the possibility of your spouse, relative or friend dying, they are by no means infallible signs. Every doctor has seen some deeply unconscious stroke patients who have made a good recovery. On the other hand, someone with a minor initial stroke may die soon afterwards from a second stroke or a heart attack.

When is the worst time?
Someone who is going to die from a stroke is most likely to die on the first day, and the risk reduces day by day, but continues for at least three weeks. The exact cause or mechanism of death varies. Some people die simply because the part of the brain necessary for maintaining breathing or heartbeat has been destroyed, others due to the sheer amount of brain tissue lost, others when the swelling that accompanies death of brain tissue presses on and destroys the brain centres that maintain breathing. A large haemorrhage is likely to cause the brain to swell and compress the vital centres.

Most people who have suffered a stroke and survived the first day probably actually die from bronchopneumonia (lung infection), which is an inevitable complication in someone who is semi-conscious. A large number die from heart disease or second strokes.

Home nursing after a stroke

First, you must see that you have the right amount of back-up. Your doctor should be able to arrange visits from a community or visiting nurse and help from support organizations (we give more details about this important aspect in Chapter 10). You should then find home care a rewarding arrangement. Not only is it often less stressful, it may also be cheaper. Some of the money saved from avoiding hospital admission might well be used to pay for specialized help for a few days or weeks. More importantly, it can be used to help alleviate any longterm disabilities: for example, you may be able to adapt a car for someone with a paralysed arm.

Should you rest after a stroke?

James Watson, a seventy year old retired butcher, had his stroke while watching television one Saturday. He lost the use of his right leg, and his right arm was clumsy. He was a bit confused, but seemed to understand what was going on around him. His daughter tried desperately to make him lie down, while he insisted on sitting up and trying to walk. She called the doctor. Mr Watson calmed down, and was cared for at home. With a little help from a physiotherapist, he was soon walking safely again.

There is no evidence that rest is of any benefit. Indeed, it is now accepted that the sooner people recovering from a stroke are moving about the better. Prolonged rest may lead to weakness and a loss of confidence, as well as other complications such as stiff joints or a clot developing in the leg veins. This is particularly true of the elderly, the people most likely to have a stroke.

There are two precautions to be remembered before someone is allowed to begin moving again. First, you must consider safety. It would be foolish to allow someone with a totally paralysed leg to try to walk without help, risking falling and injury. Similarly, it is wise to have help available the first time someone tries to use the stairs (see also Chapter 8). The answer is to provide the necessary help and not restraint. Second, if your relative has a condition associated with the stroke special rest may be needed. For example, after recovering from a heart attack people are usually advised to rest, at least for one or two days.

It is also unnecessary for someone who has had a stroke to be kept quiet. There is often an understandable feeling that someone who is ill should be protected from stress. People who have not actually stayed in a hospital may believe that this is one of the benefits of hospital care. Of course, hospitals are usually friendly places, with the staff making great efforts to relax their patients. Nevertheless, hospital life can be quite stressful – you are often woken at six o'clock; there is noise all day from cleaning machines, trolleys going up and down the ward, other patients talking; there is uncertainty as to what will happen next, the sudden appearance of a doctor; little contact with friends. It is easy to lose touch with reality in a hospital. This produces the wrong type of stress. A lively home environment, with plenty of interesting activity going on, will provide the right stimulus for recovery.

The best place for someone who has had a stroke is where there is adequate nursing care, where people will be easily able to visit, where it is comfortable and relaxing. It is unwise to keep someone isolated in a distant bedroom unless he is unconscious or it is impossible to move him. After all, no one will mind if your relative drifts off to sleep from time to time in the living room.

Are there any dietary restrictions?

Mrs Fraser, an eighty year old ex-teacher who had a stroke, was kept at home with her daughter. On the first day the nurse helped move the bed down to the living room, and provided a commode. Although severely paralysed on her left side, Mrs Fraser remained bright and cheerful, appreciating all the visits from her friends. However, she took great exception to being given rice pudding and soup when her daughter's family were eating her favourite meal of curried fish!

There is no need to give people invalid food if they can eat normally. Over the first few days about one-third of those recovering from stroke have problems swallowing. This happens more with fluids than with solids. It rarely lasts more than four to six days, and is not often a serious disability. Nevertheless, it can lead to difficulties. You may notice that the person you are nursing tends to choke when trying to swallow fluids such as tea, coffee, soup or milk with cereal. You should test swallowing with plain water (if a little enters the lungs, no harm will be done). If your relative chokes, then avoid liquid foods, particularly soups. Give frequent small drinks of water to maintain the fluid intake. Fruit gelatin (jelly) is another source of water that can be swallowed easily. Solid food should present no problems, though you should avoid crumbly food such as cake. Since the difficulty resolves itself in a few days, there is no risk of malnutrition through the low food intake. If the problem is severe, though, it is essential to get medical advice.

Besides the difficulty in swallowing, you may find that food remains in one side of your relative's mouth. Also, false teeth may suddenly seem loose. These problems are often caused by weakness of the facial muscles (this may also be the reason for slurring of speech), and should gradually get better during the recovery period.

Apart from these precautions, you should offer your relative a normal diet. Of course, once recovery is under way it may be necessary to consider longterm changes in diet. Although it is now fashionable to switch to a low-fat diet which includes some polyunsaturated fat (such as vegetable oils), there is no evidence that this will benefit anyone who has had a stroke. This diet is mainly supposed to prevent arterial disease developing in the young, and it would be unrealistic to expect much effect in anyone over sixty. There are, nevertheless, a few dietary points that should be considered:

High-fibre diet Constipation is common after a stroke because movement is so often restricted. A high-fibre diet is a better, more natural way than using laxatives to help bowel activity.

Calorie-controlled diet Being overweight makes any movement more difficult and of course this is especially true after a stroke. We recommend losing weight gradually on a calorie-controlled diet.

Adequate diet Many elderly people's normal diet is not adequate for their well-being; this is especially true of those living alone. You should encourage a diet with a protein, vitamin and calorie content that provides sufficient nourishment, according to your relative's age and level of activity.

For those who survive this early period some recovery is very likely to take place. In the next chapter we show the extent of recovery you may expect or hope for.

7 RECOVERY AFTER STROKE

The first few days after a stroke are full of action. Many practical problems have to be overcome. The patient's state often fluctuates, and many lost functions are recovered. As time goes on and the extent of mental or physical disability becomes clear, your first happiness that your relative or friend has survived can give way to worry and fear about the future. How can I cope? Will he or she walk again? How can I bathe her? Will she ever be able to talk again? In the next three chapters we hope to answer some of these worries.

The chances of survival after an acute stroke were discussed in Chapter 6. Here we describe the normal course of recovery – what exactly is recovery; who does well and who does not; what speed and how much recovery you can expect.

What is recovery and how does it happen?

Anyone who is disabled learns new ways to move or talk. This adaptation is the reason for some of the apparent recovery you may see after a stroke. Just as a man who has lost his right hand through an accident learns to shave and write using his good left hand, so someone who loses the use of an arm after a stroke can adapt. How long the adaptation takes depends upon the complexity of the action. We can all learn to feed ourselves with one hand quite quickly. Learning to dress when you can move only one arm takes much longer.

The alternative way to learn to dress is to recover some use of the paralysed arm. This recovery relies on changes beginning in the brain helping lost functions to return. In fact, the distinction between learning to adapt and recovering lost functions is artificial to a certain extent, because adaptation itself depends upon changes in the brain.

Although it has been known for centuries that many people who have had a stroke recover, the inaccessibility of the brain makes it difficult to find out how this comes about. We shall outline the various theories that are put forward.

Mrs Gertrude Foss had her stroke on May 21. She was completely paralysed on the right side and had lost all power of speech. A CAT scan (see page 44) on May 25 showed a large area of brain loss on the left side. By June 1 her speech was normal, yet she still could not walk at all, or use her right arm. She took her first steps on June 21, and one month later was walking alone using a tripod. Her arm also developed a little movement six weeks after her stroke. She returned home on July 16, and by early November she was walking to the local shops, talking normally and was able to use her right hand and arm for holding cans.

Mrs Foss's story is not unusual, and illustrates several points:

1. There was a rapid recovery over the first month, when her speech returned and leg movements started.
2. Her recovery continued, although slowly, for about six months.
3. All this happened despite the scan showing that Mrs Foss had lost a lot of brain tissue.

Dead brain cannot regenerate, yet people known to have brain loss can recover quite well. How is this? We shall look at some of the possibilities:

Processes of recovery
1. Learning new ways of coping
2. Use of other parts of the brain
3. Possible growth of nerve axons (see page 11 for a description of axons)
4. Reduction of brain swelling around the stroke area
5. Adaptation by others to the person who has had a stroke.

Learning new ways of coping is vital to a good recovery, but there may be other mechanisms at work. These have mainly been studied in animals, not human beings.

Use of other parts of the brain   This may be due to a change in the function of some nerve cells, known as plasticity. In other words, different parts of the brain somehow learn new abilities. Perhaps the brain is using previously unused or redundant pathways to transmit messages. Possibly new pathways are forged in some way. The real workings of plasticity are unknown, and we are not certain how much this occurs after stroke. It undoubtedly happens to children who have had some forms of brain damage. And it may be the most important mechanism involved in stroke recovery after the first month.

Possible growth of nerve axons Studies have shown there can be a limited amount of regrowth of damaged cells, and new growth of intact brain cells. For example, axons from intact healthy nerve cells can grow to take over space left in the nervous system. If the stroke destroyed half the axons controlling a muscle in your arm, the remaining axons might be able to sprout and control the muscle. The price paid is likely to be loss of fine control, which is a notable feature of people who have recovered from a stroke. They can no longer perform skilled jobs, such as writing, although they may have enough strength in their hand. How much this process occurs after stroke we do not know.

Reduction of brain swelling Immediately after any tissue dies, it swells with water that leaks from surrounding blood capillaries. White blood cells also enter the dead tissue. In the skull there is little space for the extra volume of the swollen brain, and so surrounding living brain is compressed. One result of this pressure is that the compressed brain stops working. It remains alive but cannot work, partly because its own blood supply is reduced. As the dead tissue is removed naturally the swelling slowly goes down.

Probably a lot of the first rapid recovery is due to this reduction of the early swelling. As the swelling goes down, the squashed brain can start to work again. This process may continue for up to eight weeks, but is usually over within two weeks.

Adaptation by others Last, and very important, we learn to adapt to the person who has suffered the stroke. Research in our hospital on recovery of speech illustrates this. A group of people who have had their speech centres damaged by a stroke have been seen for over six years. Both those with affected speech and their families thought that recovery had taken place between two years and six years after the stroke. A careful check has been kept on their speech by trained speech therapists, and they have not seen any real improvement. The families both learn to understand, and to make themselves understood better. People whose speech is impaired may also learn how to use their remaining speech more effectively.

How much recovery can you make?

It is possible to recover all the physical damage due to stroke, even if it was at first very severe.

One remarkable person we saw recently was Mr Johnson. He had retired early to lead a life of leisure. On his fifty-eighth birthday he awoke totally unable to speak. I saw him forty-eight hours later when he was bewildered, still unable to speak or understand any words, spoken or written. Our speech therapist visited him at home two days later, when he was a little better. She could not give him any therapy as he insisted that he and his wife must go on a two week coach tour they had already reserved. I next saw Mr Johnson after their trip, twenty-five days after his stroke. His speech was perfect, as was his understanding of the spoken and written word.

His case shows that rest and quiet are certainly not essential. Such a quick recovery from such a severe loss still present two to three days after the stroke is unusual, although most doctors will know of a few people like Mr Johnson.

How do you measure recovery?

This is difficult for two reasons. First, most assessment is based on fairly rough and ready guides: can you walk? Can you dress yourself – regardless of how quickly or easily this may be done? Second, the amount and the kind of loss differs enormously from person to person, so that it is difficult to make real comparisons. Here we give some idea of recovery based upon our experience of people coming to our unit. Of the people who survive three months, our own research suggests the following chances of recovery at the end of three months:

- If you were unable to walk unaided immediately after your stroke, you stand a 65 per cent chance of being able to walk alone

- If you could not dress alone immediately after your stroke, you stand a two-thirds chance of being able to do so

- If you could not feed yourself after your stroke, you stand a 54 per cent chance of being able to do so

- If you could not get out of your bed into a chair without help, you stand a 68 per cent chance

- If your arm has no movement after two weeks, you have a 14 per cent chance of regaining the use of that arm.

In other words, most people learn to get out of bed, dress and walk unaided, and about half learn to feed themselves, but few recover the use of a paralysed arm. We have recently completed a study on everyone who had a stroke in an area of Bristol, England, called Frenchay. The table below gives some detailed results from the study. It shows how long it took for people to become totally independent in various functions at various times after a stroke. For example, 76 per cent of the people were continent three weeks after their stroke.

A lot of people ask whether recovery of lost body functions happens in a certain order. Although there is no firm answer to this question, it does seem that there is a usual order of recovery of function. This is of course not unchangeable, but it may be useful to know, as a rough guide in helping your relative return to independence. Given someone who begins by being totally dependent, perhaps unconscious, after a stroke the order seems to be:

1. Ability to sit in a chair, eat alone, provided the food is cut up; at the same time, bowel control is regained

2. Beginning of control over the bladder

3. Ability to help when being moved from the bed to a chair; at the same time complete control over the bladder

4. Ability to walk with help, shave, brush hair, wash face and clean teeth, and to dress with help

Independence after a stroke based on Frenchay community study

Time after stroke	1 week	3 weeks	6 months
People assessed	561	572	494
	%	%	%
Bowels – continent	69	87	93
Urine – continent	56	76	89
Grooming	44	73	87
Lavatory use	32	61	80
Eating	32	62	77
Moving from bed to chair	30	58	81
Walking	27	60	85
Dressing	21	49	69
Stairs	20	47	65
Bathing	14	35	51

5. Not long after, the ability to get out of bed and walk alone; at the same time, eating without help, with the ability to cut food one-handed if necessary

6. If recovery continues, the next stage is attempting stairs with help

7. Dressing without help

8. Managing stairs alone

9. Finally, for someone making a good recovery, the ability to bathe alone; this level of independence is often not reached, especially since many people would have needed help before their stroke.

Recovery – how fast and for how long?

Recovery is fastest in the early days and weeks, and is much slower after one month. This seems to apply to any kind of loss after a stroke: language, memory, strength, speed of walking. Taking dressing and walking as examples, at least half of those in our study who made a full recovery did so within fourteen days after their stroke. On the other hand, some people were still recovering after thirteen weeks, and some recovered between thirteen and twenty-six weeks after their stroke.

If we consider the people who do eventually regain use of their paralysed arm, the majority begin to have some use of it between ten and twenty days and complete their recovery after fifty to seventy days. If no movement is seen in the arm after four weeks, a full recovery is unlikely. The pattern for recovery of walking is similar.

Most people probably do not recover much after six months, although they may become more competent at those abilities they do have. For instance, you may learn to walk more safely and faster. But if you could not walk at all at six months, it is unlikely that you will learn to walk again.

Of the survivors, who recovers best?

As you may imagine, the greater the loss at first, the less successful will be the final recovery. It is possible now to identify people who may do better – or worse – than expected. People who are incontinent for longer than a day or two after their stroke tend to do less well. They are less likely to walk, for example. Yet someone who is continent but cannot walk at all after one week is very likely to be able to walk in three months.

People who lose consciousness tend not to recover so well, and neither will those with a severe paralysis. People who lose the ability to see one half of space tend to have poor recoveries. Yet from our experience, while these and many other features are important, by far the simplest and best measure of who will do well is urinary continence.

People who are continent at three days usually survive and make a good recovery in terms of walking and of getting home.

The will to improve
As with all diseases, your own will to get better is one of the most important factors, even if it can't be proved that this overcomes major losses. We know of a number of people who have given up and have either died or made poor recoveries, particularly if they were admitted to the hospital. It is vital to keep on trying, always making the most of any recovery so that you can move on to the next stage. People who simply lie back and wait to get better, or to be cured, will not do as well as those who try to help themselves. One interpretation of continent people making the best recovery is that their own strong motivation stops them from allowing themselves to be incontinent.

How does therapy help recovery?

Therapy in its widest sense is all the physical and mental help given to someone after a stroke. It is given not only by therapists but also by nurses, the family and friends, and it has many aspects.

First, it prevents some of the complications mentioned earlier. For example, correct handling should reduce the risk of someone developing a shoulder pain or contractures. Next, skilled therapists can help someone to adapt: an occupational therapist can teach dressing or eating with one hand; a physiotherapist may teach someone to walk on the weak leg, and advise on the most appropriate physical aids.

Last, therapy may help retrain the brain. A lot of time is spent on trying to encourage the recovery of different abilities. This is usually done according to a particular theory. There are several underlying physical therapy, usually named after their originators (for example, Bobath and Brunnstrom). There are also various approaches to speech therapy. Although at present there is not enough evidence to show that these therapies improve upon natural recovery, they should at least encourage and help motivate someone recovering from stroke.

A new area of therapy
One new approach that has not yet been investigated fully is based upon psychological principles. It is known as prevention of learned non-use. In short, it is thought that, because early attempts to use a paralysed arm are not successful, the brain unconsciously suppresses recovery – it learns not to use the weak arm. Prevention of learned non-use encourages even the tiniest early movements of a paralysed limb, at

65

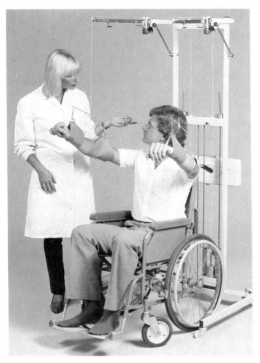

A help arm may encourage prevention of learned non-use.

the same time progressively restricting the use of the good one. In this way the sufferer is forced to learn to use the affected part.

We have seen how recovery after a stroke combines a mixture of adaptation to the loss with real recovery due to changes within the brain. This happens most quickly in the first few days and weeks, but certainly can continue for six months or more, and some people make a complete recovery. Most survivors will at least regain the ability to walk by themselves within six months. Above all, it is important not to give up; that is the way to limit recovery. In the next section of the book, we give practical advice on how relatives and friends may help immediately after the stroke, and in the long term.

8 COPING AT HOME: THE FIRST FEW WEEKS

We know of a 196 pound (89 kg) man whose stroke left him unconscious for three days, severely paralysed on his right side and without
the power of speech. His wife, registered blind and a mere 98 pounds
(44.5 kg), managed with help from the community nurse, and he
recovered well enough to potter around in his garden. In the hospital,
he may well have given up and died.

There are many other people who have recovered entirely at home,
helped by their families with assistance from various outside agencies.
Provided the family is prepared to try, to learn new techniques and not
to be discouraged when they occasionally fail, many people can be
cared for at home.

Most families are afraid that they will be unable to manage. Usually
their anxiety evaporates once they have successfully used the techniques we discuss in this chapter. Most people have no experience of
nursing or moving someone who is paralysed or bedridden and are
especially worried about this job. Clearly it is difficult for a small, frail
person to lift singlehandedly an unconscious man weighing 196 pounds
(89 kg), but the techniques we describe make even the more demanding
tasks possible.

Whether or not the stroke sufferer started by being treated in the
hospital, the problems discussed in this chapter will at some time be
faced by any relative. Of course, people admitted to the hospital have
usually made a considerable recovery before they leave. Nevertheless,
we have found about 16 per cent of people leaving our own hospital
were still needing help to get from their bed to a chair, and 24 to 30 per
cent still needed help dressing, feeding and walking.

Home care

If possible, make your first attempt at any new technique in the
presence of someone who has experience. If your relative is in the hospital, you will be taught any necessary skills before you begin home
care. For those whose relative has not been admitted to the hospital,
there are fortunately community or visiting nurses who have the right

As well as pillows for the back, it is helpful to support the arm on the weak side with pillows. This reduces the chance of the shoulder slipping out of place. The fingers should be kept as flat as possible. (*This and all subsequent photographs illustrate a stroke with weakness on the right side.*)

experience and can arrange to be present when you are trying a new skill.

The bedroom

The first consideration is where in the home you will nurse your relative. In Chapter 6 we explained why someone who is conscious but bedridden needs the stimulus of company, so that you should choose a room as close to the family's centre of activity as is practicable. If necessary, convert a downstairs room into a bedroom, bringing in all that your relative needs for comfort and to stimulate interest – a bedside light, a comfortable chair and table close by, possibly a television. At the same time, try to keep the room uncluttered and airy.

What bed?   Many people will have only their double bed available. But this is not ideal and you should try to obtain a more convenient bed for nursing.

From the invalid's point of view, a low bed is better as it is easier to get in and out. For the companion, a low bed means more bending and can lead to back problems. A single bed is much easier than a double as you can reach the person from either side. The best compromise is to move your relative to a single bed that is about 18 inches (0.5 m) off the floor.

The bed should be as firm as possible. It should have a headboard rigid enough to take the weight of someone leaning against it, and it may be useful to have a shaped back rest. Alternatively, the arrangement of pillows illustrated above should provide good support.

68

How to look after an unconscious person

It is unlikely that anyone will have to care for an unconscious person at home for more than a few days. Most people unconscious after a stroke either regain consciousness relatively soon, or they die (see Chapter 6). It is also likely that some help will be available. For example, in Britain, a district nurse will be involved, in North America, the Visiting Nurse Association or other home health agency may be able to help, and similar schemes are available in other countries. It is extremely unlikely that someone would be discharged from the hospital unconscious, and hospital admission would probably be wise if deep unconsciousness were to continue for more than a few days. The procedures we describe here would also be followed in the hospital, and even if you do not have to care for an unconscious person, it is useful to know what is done. The main principles when caring for an unconscious person are:

1. To protect the airway by keeping the head to one side

2. To move the person every two hours to prevent bed sores forming

3. Not to pull on limbs, especially the arm

4. To prevent the person becoming soaked in urine

5. To keep the mouth clean and moist.

An unconscious person is best nursed in the position shown in the illustration on page 70. He should be turned once every two hours to prevent bed sores. You should slip your arms under his body and pull him towards yourself, so rolling him over. Once turned, arrange his body and limbs in the same position as before. Keep incontinence pads in the centre of the bed and change them after turning if they are wet or soiled. Men may be kept dry by using a bottle; the penis should be placed in the spout. Women may need to have a catheter (tube) inserted into their bladder. A nurse will have to carry out this procedure but it's not likely to be needed in the first few days.

Every hour or so, swab your relative's mouth using moist lint or absorbent cotton. Every four hours, each joint should be moved gently. For example, the fingers should be gently straightened and bent, the arm straightened and bent. Feeding is not important for a few days, although liquid will be needed. Maintaining an adequate fluid intake may involve passing a tube through the nose, down into the stomach to give water or liquid food. Obviously, this is beyond your scope and a nurse will have to give the correct fluids.

If unconsciousness is prolonged, your doctor will decide on professional care.

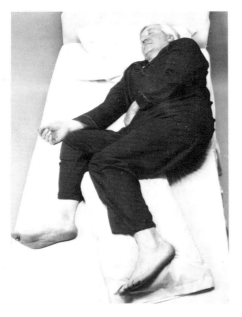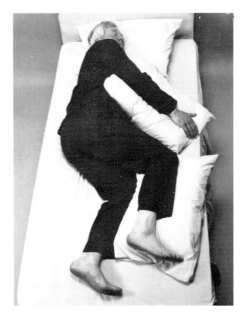

The correct positions for an unconscious person: *Left*, lying on the affected side, support should be provided by means of a pillow between the legs. The feet should be turned upwards and the upper arm placed across the body to prevent rolling back. *Right*, lying on the unaffected side, one pillow should be placed between the legs and another under the arm to support the affected shoulder.

How to look after a conscious person

Most people recover their ability to sit up unaided within a week. The tiny minority who leave the hospital still unable to sit up have probably suffered a severe stroke and not recovered fully. If that is your relative's situation, you should ask the hospital staff how to help him sit up before he comes home.

Encourage your relative to sit up in bed and take interest in the surroundings as soon as possible. Sitting up is more comfortable than lying, and it is less likely to cause choking and other problems with breathing and swallowing.

In the first few days after a stroke, your relative may find it difficult both to get into a sitting position, and to maintain it. A few people have a stroke that affects balance itself, but the usual problem is just that the paralysis on one side makes it difficult to balance. It is easiest for two people to help someone who is severely affected by a stroke to sit up. With one on each side, a cradle can be formed by linking arms under the thighs and behind the back. With a combined lift, the person can be sat

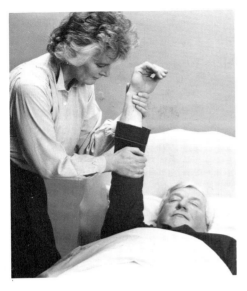
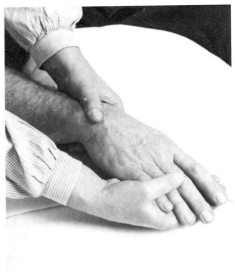
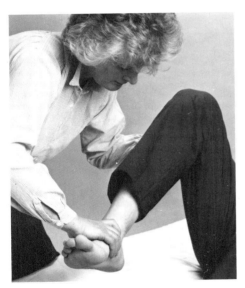
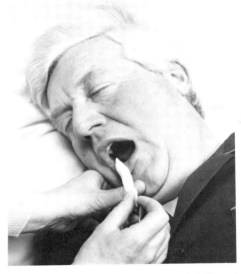

Caring for an immobile person: to prevent longterm stiffening of the joints, at regular intervals (i) raise the arms straight above the head; take care not to pull on the shoulder of the affected side (ii) straighten the fingers (iii) bend and straighten the legs. (iv) If the person is unconscious, also keep the mouth moist by swabbing it with dampened lint wrapped round a suitable instrument such as a spoon handle.

up and back against the headboard. Provide extra pillows on the paralysed side if balancing is a problem (see also the illustration on page 68).

You should also be able to lift your relative on your own, provided he or she can cooperate. You should be on the paralysed side, as shown in the illustration opposite. Place one arm around your relative's back and place his arm over your shoulder. Get him to bend his good leg up and then to push while you lift the weak side.

After a stroke, most people tend to slump towards their weak side, but it is more comfortable and safer if they can be made to sit up straight. Keep checking, and correct your relative's position as often as necessary. It should not be long before he or she can be sat out of bed in a chair.

Getting in and out of bed

No one should have to stay in bed after the first few days. But people often need helping in and out of bed for some time. Anyone admitted to the hospital will either have been taught how to get out of bed alone, or if this is not yet possible, the hospital staff should have taught you as a relative how to help.

Moving someone from bed to a chair is a hurdle that many families are afraid of, partly because it looks as if it will be difficult, and partly because they think rest is important. We should stress again that, as a general rule, mobilization is beneficial and a person who has had a stroke should get out of bed as soon as possible. As to the difficulty, we describe the method below, but it is worthwhile asking a nurse or other professional to be present if you are worried.

First place a chair, firm and not too low, near the bed (chair blocks are useful to raise low chairs and a chair with arms lends stability). Sit your relative up near the edge of the bed, then swing the legs around to hang over and touch the floor (here bed height matters). Stand on the paralysed side with one arm around your relative's back, gradually bring him forward, encouraging him to take his weight on both legs. Once standing, he should be rotated and set down gently in the chair (see the illustrations on page 74). Getting back into bed is a matter of reversing the process:

1. Stand your relative up

2. Rotate him and seat him on the edge of the bed

3. Sit him farther back into the bed

4. Swing his legs over.

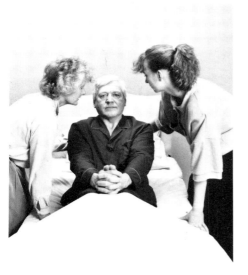 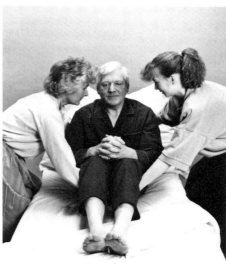

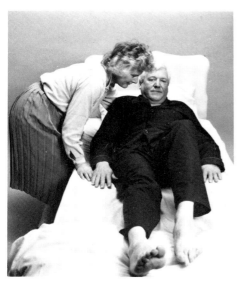 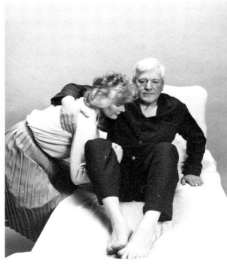

Sitting up in bed, with two people (i) raise your patient gently from the lying position (ii) link arms behind the back and beneath the thighs to form a cradle and lift carefully, taking the strain with your legs bent. With one person: (iii) lift gently from the weak side (iv) with the weak arm placed around your shoulder move the weak side back while your patient pushes with his good leg.

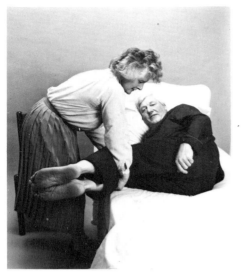
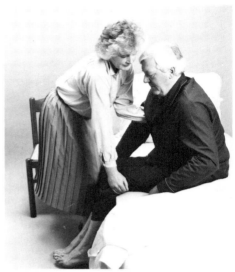
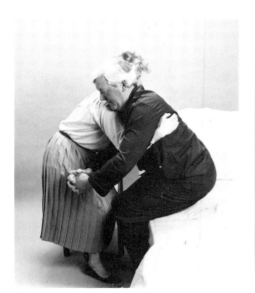
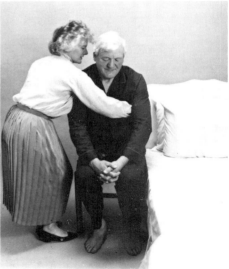

Moving out of bed (see page 72) providing support on the affected side: (i) swing the legs round (ii) raise the patient to the sitting position (iii) with the patient's hands clasped for stability, lift from beneath the strong arm (iv) rotate the patient towards the chair and seat him gently.

The important points to remember are not to pull on the paralysed arm, to have the chair correctly positioned, to remove all unnecessary clutter, and to take it slowly.

Eating

As we said in the last chapter, people usually start to eat by themselves early on in their recovery. Very few need longterm help. But you should provide appetizing food, and prepare it so that it can be eaten easily. Try to make it as nutritious as possible and give the right amount to maintain a reasonable weight. If one arm is paralysed, you will have to cut firm food such as meat and potatoes first. Use a plate with a rim so that the food is not pushed off easily, and place the plate on a non-slip mat. In this way most people can eat one-handed. Special one-handed cutlery can be a help to people who do not get back the use of their paralysed arm quickly – although we find most people prefer others to cut up their food. 'Special' aids bear a sort of stigma.

Grooming

Washing someone else is a fairly simple task. Nevertheless, there are two important points to be remembered:

1. It is vital to maintain the person's self-respect. Therefore, you should make every effort to keep your relative looking and feeling normal. False teeth should be cleaned and put in. (False teeth often no longer fit well after a stroke, and so they should be checked after three months if they feel uncomfortable.) Men should be shaved. Hair should be brushed. Women's make-up should be put on as normal.

2. Your relative should be encouraged to take on these tasks as soon as he or she can. It is demoralizing to be groomed by someone else. You should praise any attempt, but also make sure the end result is reasonable.

Although people may start to care for their personal hygiene fairly early on in their recovery, it usually takes a long time to get back to being able to bathe or shower independently. In the meantime, wash your relative all over as often as seems necessary. Your local home-nursing service should provide invaluable assistance.

Using a normal bath is a longterm problem for about half of all those recovering from stroke. As long as it is practicable and financially possible, having a shower installed is the answer. Otherwise, there are simple aids, such as non-slip bath mats, special bath seats, hand rails placed beside the bath or grab-rails attached to the taps. There are also hoists that will lift someone from a chair into and out of the bath. These come in many forms (electric, hand-powered, fixed or movable), but they are hardly ever needed by someone who has had a stroke.

Dressing

This does not often worry someone recovering from a stroke, or the family, but it often takes time. Most dressing actions need the use of both arms – putting on a shirt or sweater, doing up buttons or laces, pulling up socks and trousers – so that someone with a paralysed arm will have difficulty dressing. A few people find it hard to dress themselves even if they are not paralysed. They put clothes on back to front, or totally in the wrong place. This specific problem may be due to general confusion, and you will have to be patient. You should ask an occupational therapist to give you advice on the best way of overcoming this difficulty.

At first, family members will have to dress the person without his or her help. Take great care not to stretch any paralysed joint, especially the shoulder. Because it is important to keep someone looking normal, as far as possible dress your relative in his usual clothes.

Once the early difficulties are over, it is important to encourage your relative to dress himself, even if first efforts are slow and unsuccessful. Be patient, but be ready to help – do not allow your relative to become angry or feel defeated. Small adaptations to clothes may be necessary, but they must still look normal for your relative to want to wear them. Most people are happy to wear shoes without laces, or special one-handed laces, and women will accept Velcro fastening on their bras. Few men will want a Velcro-fastening shirt, however convenient it may be, unless it looks normal, with buttons on the front.

Starting to walk

This is often thought to be one of the most difficult hurdles, yet only 15 per cent of those recovering from stroke are left unable to walk, and most succeed without any problem.

It is best for your relative to gain confidence first by simply standing. Before suggesting walking, be sure he or she is reasonably confident about rising from a chair, standing for one minute, and then sitting down again. Next, get him to practise swaying slightly from one side to the other. He can best do this with both arms on a table to offer stability. Finally, he can start to walk. You should stand, giving support on the paralysed side while your relative make the first attempt. Give a little help in bringing the paralysed leg forward. At first, only a few steps should be tried. As with other skills, frequent short practice sessions are the most effective method of learning.

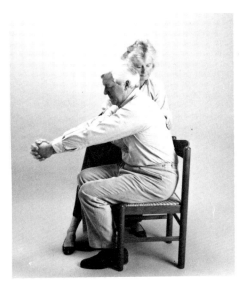
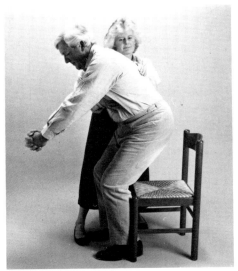
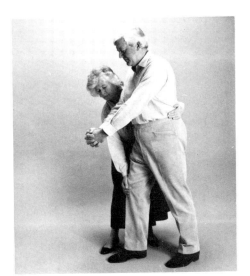
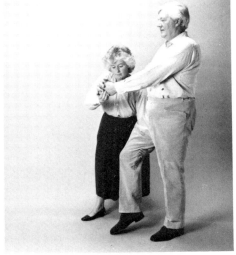

Learning to walk: (i) the arms should be held outstretched to aid stability (ii) rising to the standing position: always support the weak side (iii) keep the weak knee straight with your hand and be ready to prevent the foot slipping while the first step is taken with the good foot (iv) provide stability under the knee as the second step is taken with the weak foot.

Your relative will need to concentrate fully on walking. He will not be able to attend automatically to obstacles, such as objects on the floor, chairs in the way, sudden noises. Do make sure that there is a reasonable space to practise in. Remove any clutter from the floor; take away any small rug that may trip him; and clear away children's toys or games.

Anyone learning to walk should wear comfortable, well fitting shoes. Very loose slippers are dangerous. He must wear clothes, too, that will not get in the way.

Stairs

Once your relative is confident on his feet, climbing stairs can be considered. Nevertheless, provided getting around can be managed satisfactorily without them, it is better to delay this sort of movement until a fairly late stage. If it is necessary to get up or down stairs early on, the first safe way is to do it sitting down. Later, normal walking ascent and descent can be tried. It is slightly easier to begin by going up, but of course, you are unlikely to have the option the first time. If necessary, you should fix stair rails to the wall so that there is something to hold on

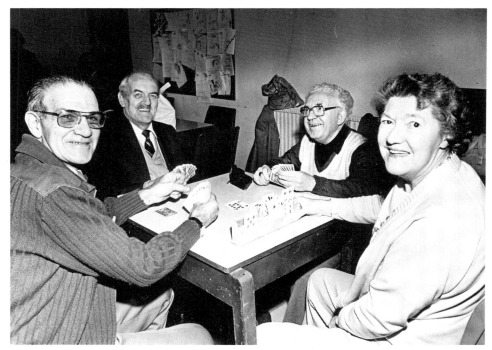

A stroke club meeting: providing encouragement and companionship which will improve the whole family's morale

to on both sides. Make sure that bannisters are secure and be at hand yourself to help.

Going out of the home
This part of getting back to normal is often the most difficult to face. Many people feel completely unable to go outside their home, not for physical reasons but for psychological ones. Your relative now has to exhibit herself to everyone, feeling and often looking abnormal, maybe unable to communicate clearly, probably much slower physically and generally feeling insecure. Some people do not recover enough to walk outside, and they should be able to be taken out in a wheelchair; but this is another barrier – who likes to be seen in a wheelchair for the first time?

It is very important to recognize this problem. It is easy to forget how unsure each of us feels even when returning to work after being ill for two weeks with influenza. Most people are ill for much longer after a stroke. They will often give reasonable excuses for not going out – 'It's too cold now', 'The street is too uneven for me', 'Next week I'll be better' – their families and other advisers often go along with their reasoning – 'Take it easy, you've got all the time in the world', 'Don't strain yourself'. The best policy is to try to prevent the problem arising by inviting visitors in during the first few weeks. This not only accustoms the person to being seen but also familiarizes the visitors with the changed person, and may encourage them to invite her out.

If it is obvious that your relative is ready to go out but does not want to, you will have to take action. One way is to encourage going out little by little, first accompanying your relative just outside the door, then to the street, then along the street a few yards, and eventually to the shops. It is best for someone to accompany your relative on these early outings. A professional helper such as a physiotherapist will be able to override all the 'medical' excuses. Alternatively, a voluntary worker may be able to persuade your relative to go out to a club or meeting for stroke victims. In our area these meetings are held in public houses, which not only increases their attraction, but also helps people regain their confidence.

Longterm help
Many people do not recover complete independence after a stroke; about half will have some longterm problems. Fortunately, it is rare for someone to be left with any severe disability simply due to a stroke. But when this does happen it is still possible for the person to be cared for at home, even though it clearly means hard work for the family. First, you have to get advice on the most efficient way of overcoming the problems. While you don't have to be expert at moving someone who is

going to recover soon, if you need to help many times a day, every day, it pays to learn from an expert how best to do it. You should also make sure that you have all the mechanical aids that can help you (see useful addresses, page 118). Most important of all, it is vital to preserve your own health. This means accepting any help available, whether from friends, voluntary organizations or commercial or public agencies. You will also need a vacation occasionally. This may be arranged by asking a hospital or nursing home to care for your relative for two weeks, or by having friends or other members of your family relieve you. These and other aspects of caring for someone after a stroke we talk about in more detail in Chapter 12.

9 LEARNING TO SPEAK AGAIN

Losing your ability to speak is one of the most feared and least understood consequences of a stroke. Fortunately, it is relatively rare to lose your power of speech or have it severely affected for a long time. We estimate that about one in ten people will be left unable to speak after a stroke. On the other hand, some disturbance of speech is very common. Probably over 50 per cent of people have some problem with speaking in the first few days. But often it is simply a brief slurring of their speech. In this chapter we will describe how you speak normally, so that you may find it easier to understand how speech can be disrupted. Then we will outline various ways of helping someone with speech problems.

Speech – a means of communication

We can communicate with each other in many ways, and speech is just one method of transferring an idea or thought from one person to another. Other ways include gestures, such as shaking your head, or making facial expressions or reading or writing.

Consider a simple everyday situation: two friends in a garden are looking at some weeds. The first says, 'I'm having terrible trouble getting rid of these weeds.' The other replies that she has some spray for killing them and goes to fetch it. On returning, she reads the instructions to herself and then tells her friend how to use the spray. The first writes down the name of the spray so that she can buy some herself later. Communication is richly developed in humans, setting us apart from other animals, and it brings together and may involve all our senses – sight, touch, smell, hearing and speaking – as well as movement and thinking.

Speech or writing

Let us look in more detail at the ways in which we communicate, starting with the generation of thoughts. We do not know how thoughts begin, although they often depend upon a sensory input: perhaps a communication from another person, an internal feeling such as

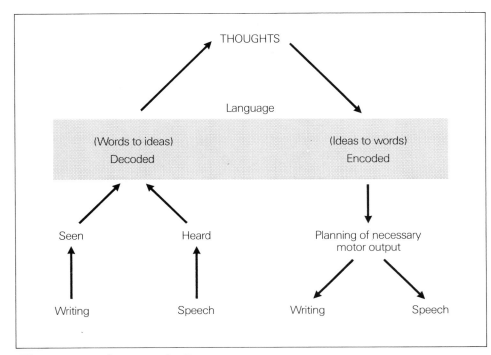

The process of communication

hunger, or an external sensation such as sight or sound of running water. Some of them you may want to let others know about.

If you have a desire to tell your thoughts to someone, they have to be put into words. This involves the use of language. In essence what is happening is a form of coding. If you smell smoke and see fire in your mind's eye, you need to find a way to let others know. Your image of fire is put into code, and that code is the word 'fire'. The sound of the word, or its written appearance, bears no relationship to real fire – it is just a convention that is termed language. Usually many words could be used, and your brain will select the most appropriate one for the circumstances; words used by young men at work, for instance, may not be used in front of their mothers, even if the underlying thought is similar!

There are various ways that the word can be transferred from one person to another. The commonest one is to use your voice, but writing is an alternative. Whatever the means, further processes need to happen before communication is halfway complete. The necessary actions are planned and then carried out in a coordinated fashion.

Speaking
If you decide to speak the word, your brain will have to work out how to make the noise 'fire'. It has to plan the coordination of breathing, the

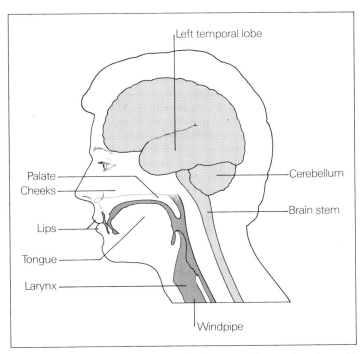

The left temporal lobe of the brain, and the speech mechanisms it governs

production of the noise by the voice box (larynx) and the modulation and control of that noise by your tongue, lips, cheeks and nose, in such a way that the correct word emerges. This planning takes place in areas of brain near the language centre in the left temporal lobe (under your left temple, see illustration above). Then more detailed coordination happens in the balance areas of the brain in the cerebellum. The final messages to the muscles come from within the brain stem (see also below).

If you decide to write, a similar process of planning and coordination takes place. Planning includes deciding which letters are needed to spell out the word. In this case the final output is usually to the arms and hands. The actual command given will depend upon whether you are using a pen or a typewriter.

Receiving the message

Once the words have left you, the speaker or writer, they need to be received, decoded and understood. The words have to be heard and listened to, or seen and read. The noises or letters need to be retained and analysed, recognized as words, and the words decoded to give the original idea. Sometimes, we may have difficulty in doing this if we hear an unfamiliar word. Interpretation (decoding) is greatly helped by the context, which often allows us to guess the meaning of unfamiliar or unclear words. This is influenced by our own experience, education and familiarity with the speaker. Finally, the ideas need to be incorporated into your thinking, and acted upon if necessary.

Which parts of the brain are involved?

Much of the brain is involved in communication, but some areas have special functions. One particular part of your brain is responsible for turning thoughts into words. In almost all righthanded people and about half of all lefthanded people, this part of the brain is on the left. It is called the left temporal lobe. In about one person in twenty the language centre is in the right temporal lobe. Decoding words, whatever their origin, takes place in the same language centre in the left temporal lobe. There is a slight separation of the two processes within the left temporal lobe, one part dealing with encoding or turning thoughts into words, the other with decoding or turning words into thoughts. The two areas are closely linked. Two other parts are particularly important. The cerebellum helps in coordinating the muscle output, whether for speech, reading or writing. The brain stem contains the nerve cells that connect with the muscles of speech.

Disorders of communication

A stroke can upset any of these processes, and may upset several at the same time. This can be very distressing to the person concerned. Even some doctors, nurses and other hospital staff are not used to distinguishing the various ways that communication can be disturbed, and may either assume people cannot understand when they can, or that they can when they cannot. We shall describe in some detail the more frequent problems and simple ways of deciding what the difficulties are. We hope you will then be able to understand what really is the problem, and so communicate more effectively with anyone whose speech is affected by a stroke. Here we list the different categories of communication difficulties:

1. Confusion

   Thoughts muddled:

   - actions inappropriate
   - speech grammatical but with inappropriate content

2. Aphasia

Loss of use of language:

- inability to find the correct word
- use of nonsense words
- speech, reading and writing affected

3. Apraxia

Inability to speak despite intact language (see page 86).

4. Dysarthria

Speech is slurred but:

- correct words are used
- understanding is unaffected
- reading and writing are unaffected.

Confusion

Many people are confused immediately after a stroke – about 30 per cent of those who have had a stroke. Confusion means that your ideas are muddled and incorrect. You are not quite sure what has happened, where you are or who you are. You may think it is summer when it is winter; that it is night when it is day; that you are at home when you are in the hospital. When the original ideas are confused, your speech reflects this and is confused too. It may be grammatical and consistent, but bears no relation to reality.

Aphasia

This is the most distressing loss that happens after stroke. The medical terms are aphasia or dysphasia. Any stroke damaging the left temporal lobe area may lead to disruption of the language centre. Ideas can no longer be converted correctly into words. You tend either not to speak at all, or to use incorrect words. A watch is called a torch, a table a mat. You may grope for words, banging your hands in frustration. Sometimes you can suddenly find a word or phrase, only to forget it on another occasion. You are also often unable to understand spoken or written words. You rely upon clues, such as someone's hand gestures. This difficulty in understanding varies from one time to another. Sometimes, particularly if the damage is mild, you may just miss certain subtleties of language, losing the precise meaning of a word or sentence. This is more likely if someone speaks to you quickly.

We all occasionally lose a word, or cannot name someone. This frustrating experience should give us some insight into the frustration felt by people with language loss after a stroke. Just as we tend to hide our inability, so do people who have had a stroke. They appear to respond normally to conversation. They will reply, 'Good morning', when greeted, and will say 'yes', from time to time. However, their speech has no content. They have lost their ability to encode and decode. It is important not to be misled by first impressions.

Apraxia

A rare complication is the inability to plan the necessary actions to transmit the words, whether by speaking or writing. This problem is known as apraxia. A person with apraxia can find the right word but cannot recall the sounds necessary to make it. In terms of speech, he or she may speak clumsily, faltering and using incorrect sounds in the middle of words. In terms of writing, words may be spelled wrongly or letters not formed properly.

Dysarthria

A very common problem after stroke is slurring of speech. The medical term is dysarthria. This occurs when the control of your tongue, palate and lips is disturbed so that you cannot execute the movements you have planned correctly. This may happen after stroke affecting the brain stem or a cerebral hemisphere; exactly how we do not know. People with slurred speech are able to use language correctly, and can understand everything. Nevertheless, they often sound odd and may be difficult to understand. As long as their arm is unaffected, they can write normally.

Hearing and sight

Though deafness is common among elderly people who have had a stroke, it is very rarely an effect of the stroke. Complete blindness is also rare after a stroke, but loss of one half of vision can make reading difficult. This will happen if the stroke affects the side of the brain where the visual cortex lies (see the diagram on page 10).

How do I tell what is wrong?

From the companion's point of view, the first step is to be aware of these possible disturbances of communication. In particular, you should remember that about one-third of people with weakness of the right side have language disturbance. On the other hand, it is rare for people with weakness of the left-sided limbs to develop significant language problems. Confusion is common but shortlived. Slurred speech is also common. Knowing this, listen to and talk with your friend and ask yourself the following questions:

1. Is he using all his usual aids?

2. Is his understanding of speech intact?

3. Can he name objects?

4. Does he use normal sentences?

5. Does he make up nonsense words?

6. Is he confused?

Is he using all his usual aids? It is most important that anyone who needs them is wearing his glasses, false teeth and hearing aid, otherwise you will have a false impression of the effects of the stroke. Even when dentures are worn, they may be loose due to a weakening of the face muscles. In that case denture fixative can make speech clearer.

Can he understand simple questions or commands? The best test is to ask your relative or friend to perform some simple tasks. It is important not to give any clues to the answer by the way you ask or by your facial expression. You could ask the person to put his left hand on his head, to pick up some nearby object using his left hand, or to use his left hand to cover his right eye. You could ask him to point to items in the photographs in a newspaper or magazine. He should be asked to use his left hand because the right arm will probably be paralysed if there is any language disturbance. Obviously if the left hand were paralysed, the right hand should be used, though in that case it would be unusual for language to be affected.

Can he name objects? This is most easily tested by your asking the person what various items are called. Use clearly visible and familiar objects such as a pen, a watch, a cup. If the person gives the right names, press for more detail. For example, ask him to name the handle of the cup, the top, clip and nib of a pen, or the parts of a watch (hands, strap).

Does he use normal sentences? If your friend or relative can understand speech and name objects, then you can look for more subtle disturbances, which are also very important. To do this listen carefully to his speech. You may need to prompt him by asking him to tell you about his day. Check the length of his sentences: are they shorter than usual? Listen to the order of the words and phrases: does he get them muddled? Consider the words he uses: are they the ones he would normally use?

Does he make up nonsense words? A good clue to language disturbance is the use of nonsense words. These may sound correct, but actually have no meaning: 'We had fried splotic for lunch today.' The word splotic sounds like a noun, but does not exist. But make sure that the person is not simply mispronouncing a normal word. For example, if he said 'fried fizz', he might be saying 'fried fish' with a slur. Usually the nonsense word is said clearly and in a normal voice. If you ask for it to be repeated, the person will do so emphatically, as if its meaning were obvious, whereas the person with dysarthria will realize that you are having difficulty understanding and may try other words. If someone uses nonsense words you may think he's confused, but this is not often so. A confused person tends to use normal language.

Is he confused?   You will have difficulty trying to determine anything from these tests if your friend or relative is confused. You need to decide: does he know who he is, who I am, where he is and roughly the date and time. Is he behaving in his usual manner? Listen carefully to his speech. Are the sentences normal? Does what he is saying make sense? If you can understand the ideas, but they are nonsensical, he is probably confused. His behaviour will probably supply the answer. A confused person is often restless and talks about the past. Given an object such as a cup of water, a confused person will often not know what to do with it.

Provided you know that your friend or relative is not confused and that his language centre is working, you can pay attention to the way he is pronouncing his words. Slurred speech is common immediately after a stroke, affecting about 60 per cent of people. It is usually not very severe, and is shortlived. One common cause is because the person is not wearing false teeth (see above). No tests are needed to detect slurring – you can hear it. The main point is not to mistake slurred speech for confusion and lack of understanding. However, you should test swallowing. Ask your relative to try and drink some water. If he or she chokes, you must take care with feeding (as mentioned on page 57). Food also may tend to dribble out of the corner of his mouth.

To recap: many people have slurred speech after a stroke, so that they sound a bit drunk, and many are confused. Both these states are usually shortlived. It is especially important to recognize confusion. Confused people are restless and their speech makes sense but is not sensible. People with aphasia on the other hand have a specific problem with the use of language – this may affect speaking and understanding. You can discover which problem your relative has using the tests we described above.

Being aware of the ways communication can be disturbed, and using these simple tests should help you identify the problem. However, we feel that anyone with obvious speech disturbance lasting over two weeks should be assessed by a professional speech therapist or speech-language pathologist. She will offer advice and treatment initially, but the most important people in the long term are friends and relatives. It is their continual encouragement and stimulation that is vital in helping the sufferer overcome his problems.

Talking to someone affected by stroke

First, the practical advice we have given already is again essential here. Being unable to see or hear properly – especially after the shock of a stroke – can be a major cause of confusion. See that your relative or friend is in a quiet, well-lit room wearing his glasses, false teeth and hearing aid, before you begin to talk with him. Next, remember that the best way you can help someone with speech difficulty is to provide encouragement and stimulation. Most people recovering from a stroke become very depressed or frustrated by their difficulty. They may be embarrassed, demoralized or humiliated. It is essential for them to keep trying to speak.

Confusion

If you are trying to communicate with someone who is confused, make sure that the surroundings are not distracting (see also below). Keep the conversation simple. Fortunately, confusion usually lasts only a few hours or days.

Aphasia or apraxia

People with these disabilities need encouragement to use whatever speech they have. Unfortunately, many people withdraw into themselves, avoiding any conversation. They need to be given reasons that will increase their desire to talk. For example, showing photographs of familiar places or people, discussing vacations, or gossiping about friends. Obviously, this can be time-consuming but devoted attention is the most valuable aid to somebody with language impairment.

If your relative has any of those language disturbances we listed under aphasia (page 84), then the main rule is to use short, simple sentences, and speak clearly and slowly. How simple you make your language will obviously depend on your relative's level of understanding. You may obtain some guidance on the best approach from a speech therapist. As this is not always possible in the first weeks after the stroke, we also provide some general guidelines.

You should try and reduce any distracting noises; turn off the television or radio and speak clearly and slowly using short, simple sentences. There is no advantage in speaking loudly, except to deaf people. Use gestures and mime to help with your speech. Give your relative time to understand. Wait before each new sentence, or repeating yourself. Avoid complicated ideas if at all possible. Remain interested, and do not appear impatient. Encourage your relative, and help him find the correct word. Treat him as an intelligent adult, not an imbecile.

Someone with aphasia will also tire easily. It is obviously a time-consuming effort to maintain this level of concentration for a long period. Therefore, space out attempts at communication. But it is vital not to talk across people with language disturbance as if they were not there. First, it is rude and humiliating. Second, they often do not understand much of the conversation, and may well misinterpret some of it. It is, though, reasonable to talk in their presence to someone else without necessarily including the person who is aphasic, provided you make it clear that they are part of the conversation in spirit if not in fact.

Dysarthria

People often assume that someone with slurred speech is in some way mentally defective. He is not, and is fully able to understand. Assuming language function is normal, you may talk normally. Your relative's speech will usually be intelligible provided you concentrate and there is not too much background noise. You should encourage him to talk slowly and to avoid long words that are difficult to pronounce. People with slurred speech are rarely so badly affected that they need help with reading or writing. But if someone has persistent badly slurred speech which makes him impossible to understand, he may need to communicate by writing or using aids (see page 92).

Professional help

Your most important helper is a speech therapist or speech-language pathologist. If you have to wait for a couple of weeks before seeing one, it will not be time lost, especially as so many people recover on their own during this period. On the other hand, some people and their families are so anxious at this time that early attention from a speech therapist is a great comfort. The practical consideration of the availability of qualified therapists often determines when you may first see one. In any case, your doctor should advise your relative to see a therapist if the speech problems continue after two weeks.

How a speech therapist can help

1. Diagnose precisely what is wrong

2. Explain what is wrong

3. Advise on the best way of communicating

Rules for helping someone with language problems

1. Allow time for understanding and to talk; do not hurry him
2. Speak slowly and clearly at a normal volume
3. Use familiar words in short sentences
4. If necessary, repeat using different words
5. Gestures, not too exaggerated, often help
6. Never underestimate your relative's comprehension, but realize that he may have difficulties
7. Avoid long, rambling conversations
8. Do not change the subject too quickly
9. Encourage all his attempts
10. Be prepared to help him find words, and encourage him to repeat them
11. Expand his brief utterances; for example, if he says 'lavatory', say, 'Do you want to go to the lavatory?'
12. Never pretend to understand if you do not
13. Do not expect as much as usual if he is tired or emotionally upset
14. Remember he is easily distracted
15. Do not ask others questions he can answer
16. Talk to him while performing other activities, such as teaching him other skills
17. Involve him in all routine activity
18. Discuss his problems with him
19. Remember, he is an intelligent adult.

4. Give treatment
5. Contact local voluntary support groups
6. Check progress.

The therapist's first job is to establish the nature of the problem. To do this he or she will probably use special tests that take anything up to one hour to complete. She will also discover which parts of language function and speech production are still intact. She will then be able to explain to the family exactly what their relative can and cannot do. This will help them communicate better with each other. If slurring is the major problem, the therapist should give advice on the best way to make speech more understandable. Aids which may help people with slurring are usually no use to those with aphasia. Nevertheless, most therapists believe that speech therapy can help in the recovery of the power of speech. To be really effective, therapy for these conditions should be given for more than the customary few hours a week. It is here that help from family and friends, with the guidance of the therapist, is all-important.

Support groups

By introducing the family to voluntary support groups the therapist will extend the benefit of her advice. The type of help offered by these groups varies. Sometimes it is more or less formal 'therapy', an attempt at retraining some aspect of speech such as the ability to name simple objects. At other times a volunteer will stay with the stroke victim while the family goes out shopping, or will take him to a special group for people with language loss. The therapist should always be consulted about the part the voluntary group should play.

The last role of the therapist is to monitor recovery. Most people make some recovery of their speech and this means that the family will have to change their approach as time goes by. The therapist should see that the family is aware of the recovery and make full use of it. For someone with severe dysarthria, the therapist will also need to check that appropriate techniques and aids are being used.

Can artificial aids help?

There is a wide variety of aids available, including boards with pictures to point at, typewriters attached to television screens or printers, computers and even artificial voices. These are very useful for people who have an undamaged language centre but are unable to speak or write normally. People left with severe speech disturbance after a stroke have usually lost their language centre so that the aids are useless to them. The majority of people with speech disturbed by a stroke do not need aids of any kind. Time and therapy provide their recovery.

Further assistance for all types of disabilities from outside helpers and agencies is important in the long term. In the next chapter we give some useful information about where you may seek help.

10 WHO CAN HELP?

So far we have concentrated on how you manage at home if you or a relative has had a stroke. We have also mentioned that there is help available from various sources outside the home. There is a wide range of aids and services for the physically handicapped and these we describe in this chapter. Allowing for variations in the fine detail, equivalent services exist in the UK, North America, Australia and other Western countries. The differences are mainly concerned with who pays for them.

Immediate help – your doctor
Your family doctor is likely to provide the first professional help you call on. He or she will have a vital role to play over the whole course of the illness. He will first make a diagnosis and decide whether you (or your relative) should be admitted to the hospital for further tests or treatment, or should attend as an outpatient. Alternatively, he may ask a hospital specialist to see you at home.

Your doctor will be able to offer two other types of assistance. First, and most important, he will probably explain exactly what has happened, what is likely to happen and what he proposes to do. This information should also be given to you by any of the doctors you see if you are admitted to the hospital. You should not be afraid to ask questions. Most doctors are happy to answer them; they just sometimes forget to offer information. Do not worry about asking apparently stupid questions – if they worry you, then they are important. Do not be afraid to ask the same question again later, we all forget 90 per cent of answers given by our doctors! Write down questions as you think of them, before seeing the doctor.

Your doctor is also your main source of information about any practical help you need. He should know either whom to approach directly or where to find further information. When he first comes to see you, he will need to discuss with you and the rest of the family whether or not you would prefer home or hospital care. If you prefer home care, then he will organize any nursing help needed.

Nursing help

The most important early home help is usually given by the district or visiting nurse. These are highly skilled home nurses and in our opinion they are capable of caring for any stroke patients at home, given the right additional support from the family.

Mrs Emily Sharp, aged eighty-nine, lived with her seventy year old daughter in a small town. She had her stroke while getting dressed one morning, and immediately became unconscious. Their family doctor was called and diagnosed a stroke. Although the daughter had arthritis, she wished to nurse her mother at home. Two community nurses called within an hour and got Mrs Sharp back into bed. Mrs Sharp regained consciousness but remained almost helpless. Nevertheless, with the help of the nurses she was able to stay in her own home. Over her last few days, they called three times each day for fifteen minutes, helping bathe, turn and feed Mrs Sharp. She died peacefully seven days after the stroke.

So there are few obstacles to home care, provided that it is what is wanted. The daughter herself was disabled, and the old house apparently unsuitable with narrow stairs and no running water upstairs. Nevertheless, with frequent but short visits by the nurses, Mrs Sharp was nursed successfully at home.

The District or Visiting Nurse should be contacted as soon after the stroke as possible, and this is best done by the doctor. She can arrange for a commode to be provided (a portable lavatory, usually in the form of a chair), help move a bed to the best place, and move the patient to the bed. She can show you how to move, feed and wash your relative, and she can visit as often as is necessary.

At the beginning, she will call daily, both to teach the family how to nurse their sick relative and to do some nursing herself, particularly washing the patient. Later she will help get your relative out of bed into a chair, and then walking around. She will arrange other help: as well as a commode, a hoist or walking sticks may be needed. She can arrange for a home help, Meals-on-Wheels and other services (see also page 118).

Your District or Visiting Nurse can:

● Help nurse dependent people

● Provide immediate aids (such as a commode)

● Help rearrange the house

- Teach you how to handle someone with a stroke
- Refer you to other agencies
- Provide emotional comfort.

If for some reason your doctor forgets to arrange help, then you should be able to contact a nurse directly via the social services. If extra help is needed, look into the possibility of private nursing care for a few hours a day; although this is expensive, it may be needed for only a few days. Nursing agencies usually advertise in telephone directories, newspapers and so on, but your doctor will also know how to contact them. Sometimes free extra help may be available from charitable organizations.

In those countries without state-provided community nursing, there are many nursing agencies (for example, the Visiting Nurse Association in the USA), which can provide similar services. While nursing care is expensive, it is almost certainly cheaper than hospital care. Constant nursing is not necessary.

Therapy
Later on, your doctor may suggest physiotherapy, or other therapy. As we have seen, this is not necessary immediately since so many people recover by themselves. Physiotherapists get people walking and suggest which are the most suitable walking aids – canes, Zimmer frames or walkers, foot splints. They also have an important role to play in getting movement back into paralysed arms. Occupational therapists train you to dress and cook for yourself during your recovery. We talked about speech therapy in Chapter 9. You will probably have to attend the hospital for speech therapy sessions.

Therapists can:

- Make a skilled assessment of the main problems

- Show you how to handle someone correctly, reducing the possibility of complications

- Supervise first attempts at any movement of paralysed limbs

- Teach people who have had a stroke how to manage with their disability

- Teach helpers how to be most helpful

- Give exercises and advice that will encourage recovery

- Give advice on the most useful aids

- Give emotional support.

The distinction between physiotherapy and occupational therapy varies from hospital to hospital and from country to country. Occupational therapists who visit people at home often have to concentrate on authorizing costly aids and do not have much time to spend on teaching. Instead, occupational therapy such as advice on dressing may be given by the district nurse visiting your home, while retraining for work, whether housework or paid employment, will mean attending the hospital.

In Britain therapists are usually based in hospital departments. In other countries they may be contacted through special agencies that your doctor should be able to tell you about. For example, in the USA the Visiting Nurse Association, the National Easter Seal Society for Crippled Children and Adults, or other home health agencies may all be able to help.

Another way of getting expert advice is to attend the local hospital as an outpatient. Again, your doctor will probably have to ask for you to see the therapists. But this is not an ideal arrangement for everyone. You may not be fit enough to be transported there and back; often there is a long waiting list for an appointment and by the time you get any advice, it may be too late to be of any use. Then the therapist will not be able to give as much help with any particular obstacles you may have in your home environment.

Does home therapy work?

Many people, including doctors and therapists, wonder whether effective therapy can be given at home. After our recent two-year study of home care after an acute stroke, we are convinced that it can. Our physiotherapist was converted. She found she was never restricted in the type of therapy she could give. The lack of some of the more traditional equipment, such as tilting beds and parallel bars to learn to walk between was more than compensated for by the therapy being more relevant to people's particular needs. People were generally more relaxed and happier than those she had been treating in the hospital. The occupational therapist, too, found the close involvement of the family made her help more effective.

Our home care speech therapist was asked to see a lot of people she would not have seen in the hospital. Many had shortlived or minor disturbances of speech. She spent time simply giving advice on how to

96

cope as recovery occurred naturally. When giving therapy, she found it just as easy at home as in the hospital.

So therapists can easily assess and treat people at home. If you want this, it is best to ask your doctor first, as in theory at least therapy is prescribed by a doctor. Otherwise you could ask your nurse to put you in touch with a therapist.

Social services and community services

In most countries a number of services are available to people at home. In the UK some are completely free; for others there is an enquiry into your financial state and some people have to pay a contribution towards the cost.

Help around the house is available daily if needed. Helpers can clean, make beds, do the shopping, collect prescriptions and generally help run the house. Home help is usually provided by the Social Services in the UK. In the USA these services may come from a family service agency, a homemaker-home health aide agency, or a home-health agency. Such help can be invaluable both in the short term, to free the other members of the family so that they can care for the person with the stroke, and in the long term.

Other services are Meals-on-Wheels, cooked meals delivered six days a week, and day centres or day care clubs. These are places where disabled or infirm people are looked after for most of the working day. In some, therapy and nursing care, such as bathing, is also offered; other centres may be more concerned with industrial retraining. Some of these centres are based in the hospital, others in the local community. You probably won't need a day centre in the early stages of recovery – they are more suitable for people with a longterm disability.

Voluntary services

These provide enormous comfort, support and encouragement. Joining local self-help groups and societies will show you and your relative how many others have similar problems to yours, and sharing your experiences with people who really understand what you've been through should help you in the long term far better than trying to cope in isolation. For directories listing the many organizations available to disabled people, see Further Reading, page 117.

There are so many that it's obviously impossible to give names of all in the confines of this book. In order to find out about what kind of local services exist you can also:

1. Ask your doctor, nurse and therapist

2. Ask social workers, who usually know of most local support groups; they may be contacted either in the hospital or in local community offices

3. Ask any friends who have had a stroke themselves

4. Ask your local minister

5. Ask your national stroke association; they will know most local support groups and probably have one of their own.

Of the many agencies, some help only people suffering from a stroke, others help anyone disabled, yet others may be limited to special groups (for example, those unable to speak, or those under sixty-five years). Some concentrate on providing physical aids such as wheel-chairs, others give personal support. Some offer special facilities, for example, fishing for the disabled.

Physical aids

Commodes
The great advantage of a commode is that it is easy to use. The disadvantages are that some people object to having a commode permanently next to their bed, and it has to be emptied often. Alternative means of toileting do exist. For urination, a man can use a bottle; both men and women can have a tube (catheter) inserted into the bladder to drain the urine. Bedpans are less useful. Anyone who can be seated on a bedpan and can balance there could almost certainly manage more easily on a commode.

Since at the beginning the sick person's state may change so rapidly, it is better not to obtain any other special aids. After the first few days, you can start to consider what may be needed. But you will always have to balance the advantages of any aid against the chances of it not being wanted for long.

Hoists
A completely immobile person can be moved from the bed to a chair and in and out of the bath with a hoist (see the illustration opposite). There are both mobile hoists that can be operated by a hand crank and fixed hoists that can be powered by electric motors. Very few people

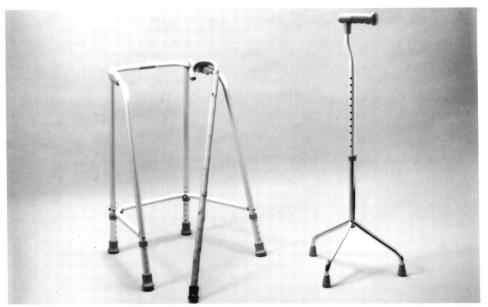

Above, recommended walking aids for people who have had a stroke. A Zimmer frame, walking stick and tripod.

Below left, a bath seat, *right* a hoist for less mobile people.

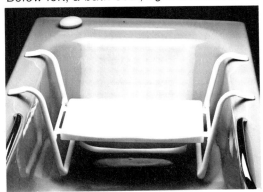 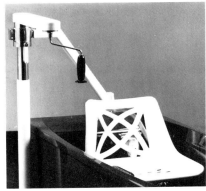

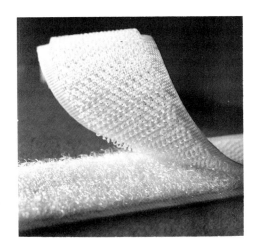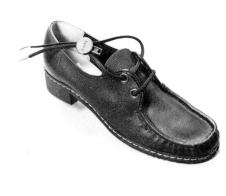

Left, Velcro is an invaluable fastening for people who can use only one hand. *Right*, shoelaces can be tightened with one hand with this simple device.

recovering from a stroke remain so immobile that they need a hoist for a long period, and so there is hardly ever any point in trying to obtain a hoist.

Mobility aids

There are many simple, cheap aids to help you move about, and these are mostly worth having, though do take professional advice about their suitability, and the correct way to use them. For example, a Zimmer frame or walker may appear to be a good way to help people to walk (see the photograph on page 99). Although this is sometimes true, some doctors and therapists think that a Zimmer frame may actually hold up recovery. It can increase a person's dependence upon firm support. A more important, practical problem is that people with a paralysed arm are unable to hold the frame – this severely restricts its usefulness. Even a walking stick is frowned upon by some physiotherapists, although our view is that anyone should feel free to use one if it gives confidence. Other common aids include various supports designed to prevent the foot from stumbling, tripods and rolling walking aids.

There are a lot of other aids to mobility. First, and most obvious, is a wide range of wheelchairs. Some are self-propelled, some need to be pushed and some are electrically powered. Some are suitable for indoor use, others for outdoor use. Some can be folded easily to go into a car. Although over 80 per cent of those who recover from a stroke regain their ability to walk, many people can still get some benefit from a wheelchair, for example, to be pushed to the shops. In Britain, the Artificial Limb and Appliance Centres (ALAC) supply wheelchairs. You need your doctor's authority to be supplied with one. They can also be bought privately, which is the usual way of obtaining a chair in the USA (although Medicare or Medicaid will supply one free if you qualify). Before you decide on a wheelchair, it is best to wait until it is clear what level of mobility you are going to reach. This should be after about four to six months. It is also essential to obtain expert, unbiased advice on the best type for you. Your therapist is the person most likely to be able to help.

Aids around the house
There are several alterations and additions that can transform your mobility inside the house. Stair rails can make it safe to go up and down stairs. It is possible, but expensive, to fit a stair lift. In the UK these may be provided on loan by the Social Services. In other countries they will have to be bought, and again you should obtain unbiased advice from your therapist before spending large sums of money – you might also consider moving into a new house.

Single steps can prove to be impossible obstacles, particularly for someone in a wheel chair. And a lot of people have to go up or down steps to get in and out of their house. These difficulties can be overcome with either a concrete ramp or removable wooden ramp. Again, in the UK the Social Services can help.

Personal and domestic aids
There are many devices designed to help you to be independent: one-hand shoelaces, aids for one-handed feeding, and non-slip mats that stabilize plates for people paralysed on one side; egg-cups that can be attached to the table. You can also replace buttons with Velcro fastenings. Despite the range, in our experience few people who have had a stroke actually use these aids. This may be for several reasons. Some are too complicated. Others are too obviously abnormal, and embarrass the user; who would wish to be seen drinking out of a baby cup? Often it is easier for a friend or relative to help rather than to use an aid: your spouse or relative can cut up food and do up buttons and shoelaces.

Which aid is for you?
Although a lot of people do not like using aids that look ungainly, (for example, large-handled cutlery), it is always worth considering anything that might help. This can be done in several ways:

101

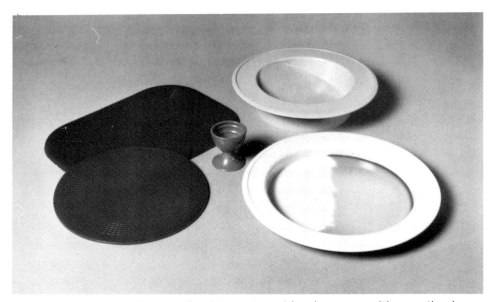

Eating aids, left to right, non-slip plate mats, a ridged egg cup with a suction base, a sloped bowl and a less obviously sloped plate; the latter is more acceptable and still helps one-handed feeding.

1. A local professional, usually an occupational therapist, may be able to give you advice.

2. You can go to a shop specializing in aids and ask the staff. They often give good advice, even though they have an interest in selling.

3. You can go through a day or two asking yourself whether you feel that a particular aid might help. Then you need to discover whether any such aid exists. Ask your therapist, your friends or a shop selling aids for the handicapped.

Who supplies aids?

As we have mentioned, aids can be obtained from a variety of sources, depending upon the kind, where you live and your financial state. In the UK most are available on free loan from the state, either through your local doctor or from the Social Services department of your local authority. You may need to make a contribution towards some aids. In every country there are charitable organizations that will lend equipment. These include the local Red Cross, local stroke associations and other special groups. Your doctor, nurse or therapist will know of the locally active agencies. Other equipment usually has to be bought commercially.

In conclusion, we want to reinforce what should be your main objectives in obtaining aids:

1. Balance the expense of obtaining an aid against the time that it is likely to be needed, taking into account the natural recovery over the first few months.

2. Decide whether the aid will really be used, however sensible it might appear.

3. Always try to obtain expert and unbiased advice.

4. It is best to approach your local Social Services department first for both free advice, and often the aid itself.

5. Decide whether any voluntary organization or special charity can give advice, and can give or lend the aid, at least on trial.

Can an operation help?

In some hospitals people with longterm problems have an operation for their disability, but in most, operations are shunned altogether. There is no agreement in the medical profession as to whether operations to help longterm disability are effective. You will have to take the advice of your doctor and specialist on this question, based on their knowledge of the success rate of such an operation.

In this chapter we have tried to give an idea of the range of services and aids that are available to patients disabled by a stroke. It is impossible to give specific detailed advice as local and personal circumstances vary so much. But do ask for help from your doctor. He or she can usually arrange for any necessary services, and tell you about others for specialized advice on aids.

11 LIFE AFTER STROKE

Live each day to the full, as if it were your last. This advice, given to the healthy, applies equally to those who have had a stroke. There is no reason why you should not do anything that you wish within your capability. In fact, you should make it your goal to get back as closely as possible to your former lifestyle. Naturally, there are questions that you would like answered. We will look at some of them now.

Might I have another stroke?
The risk of another stroke is, quite naturally, probably the main worry everybody has who has recovered from a stroke. As we mentioned in Chapter 3, the fact that you have had a stroke cannot prevent you having another. Indeed, your risk is slightly increased. An estimated 10 per cent of those who survive will have another stroke within a year. On the other hand, and more optimistically, 90 per cent of those who recover from stroke will not have one in the following year.

Perhaps more important, you actually stand a greater risk of developing heart trouble than having a further stroke. More stroke survivors die from a heart attack or heart failure than from a stroke, though this could be many years afterwards. Of course, death must come to all of us and it has to be faced that someone who has suffered a stroke does have a reduced life expectancy compared with his or her contemporaries.

Can I reduce the risk of a stroke?
To reduce your chances of having a stroke, either a first or subsequent one, we would offer the following advice:

1. Keep fit and active, and stop smoking

2. Lose weight if necessary

3. Have your blood pressure checked and treated if necessary

4. Taking an aspirin a day might help (see page 105).

While it has not yet been proved that any of these measures (apart from control of high blood pressure) necessarily reduces your risk of a stroke, they certainly will not increase it and they should improve your general health. If you have already had a stroke, they will improve your ability to manage with whatever disability you may have. They should too, reduce your risk of developing heart trouble, particularly if you stop smoking.

What part does your doctor play?
Your doctor can help reduce your risk in three ways:

1. Most importantly, he or she can check your blood pressure and treat it if needed. He should also check whether you have any other underlying cause of stroke, although this is unlikely. We frequently recommend that people's blood is checked for anaemia (too few red blood cells) and polycythaemia (too many red blood cells), as this may be the cause of a thrombosis (see Chapter 3). Your doctor should also check whether you have diabetes.

2. He should enquire into your lifestyle and give you advice on how to stop smoking, lose weight if necessary and keep active.

3. He may consider drug treatment. Unfortunately, the evidence so far is that drug treatments – except those for lowering high blood pressure – have not been beneficial for most people who have had a stroke. Some doctors give drugs designed to reduce the clotting ability of your blood (anticoagulants such as warfarin). These drugs do not help most people, and they do carry risks (see page 48). The only possible exception is aspirin, which may help some people, particularly men aged sixty-five or less. One adult tablet or less per day is unlikely to do any harm, and may reduce your risk of a heart attack or stroke.

Should I restrict my activities?
No. Definitely not. There is no logical, medical reason for you not to do whatever you wish and are able to do, within reason. Obviously, certain activities may be impossible or ill-advised. Rock-climbing with a paralysed arm would be difficult and risky. Otherwise, you should be as active as you wish – and a little more so.

Various well-meaning people may give different advice. One common warning is that you should avoid lifting heavy weights or straining yourself physically. There is no evidence that either of these is harmful. Another activity often warned against is bending; some people say you should not bend down, others that you should not look up! Neither precaution is sensible. Other suggestions we have heard include avoiding digging, not drinking alcohol, not worrying (as if that were possible) and not travelling by air. Apart from drinking excessive alcohol, you may do all of these.

What about sex?

There is no medical reason for restricting or changing sexual activity after a stroke. Obviously many people do, for several reasons. First, physical disability itself may make sexual intercourse more difficult than before. This is probably the easiest problem to overcome. There are alternative positions and methods, some of which are described in Dr Christine Sandford's *Enjoy Sex in the Middle Years*, in this series. For anyone paralysed by a stroke, it is usually much easier to make love if you lie on your weak side. This leaves your unaffected arm free. Most people devise their own solutions once they realize that this is safe.

A more difficult problem is loss of interest or desire. This may affect either the person who had the stroke or the partner. (If both no longer wish to continue sexual activity, obviously you have no problem.) The stroke victim may lose desire for sex as part of a depressive illness, or because genital sensation is decreased, or possibly as a side effect of drugs prescribed; some drugs for high blood pressure, for instance, decrease sex drive. Someone may lose the desire for sex because his or her partner no longer appears physically attractive. Serious illness in one partner can cause stress in an already frail marriage. This may lead to the stroke being used as an excuse for no longer continuing sexual activity and may sometimes even lead to divorce, although this is unlikely.

In order for desire to be restored, it is important for you to seek out the cause. This means that you and your partner should discuss the problem openly together, as well as taking advice from your doctor. Apart from avoiding drugs thought to reduce sexual ability or drive, there is little that can be done with medical treatment – that does not help. But, don't be afraid to discuss the situation with your doctor: he should be able to refer you to someone who specializes in sexual difficulties.

What about driving?

Legally, in Britain at least, you are required to:

Tell the Drivers Medical Branch, DVLC, Swansea SA1 1TU, at once if you have any disability (this includes any physical or mental condition) which affects (or may in future affect) your fitness as a driver if you expect it to last more than three months.

106

If you still have a fair amount of disability three months after a stroke, or if you have had any epileptic fits at all, clearly you should inform the licensing authorities. They often allow people to drive provided they are satisfied that you are physically and mentally safe. It is also necessary to inform your insurance company. If they or you are unsure as to your ability, or if you wish to take advice, you should ask a driving instructor to assess you. The assessment will test your fitness to drive and should provide information on any adaptations you may need to make to your car.

Depression after a stroke
You should not feel you are unusual if you suffer some depression. At least one-third of all those recovering from a stroke feel depressed and unhappy. This is mainly due to the shock of being disabled – it is a psychological reaction to the sudden severe illness and may also be a reaction to a restriction on your social activities. There is also a tendency for people who have had a stroke, or any other serious illness for that matter, to be more emotionally unstable so that they cry very easily. We know of a lot of people who can no longer watch the television news because there is usually some item that causes them to burst into tears. But emotional control usually returns.

Overcoming depression
It is not easy at the best of times to overcome depression, and it is probably especially difficult to conquer after a stroke. Treatment with such drugs as nortriptyline can help anyone with truly persistent depression. But these drugs have side effects and are unlikely to be the best solution for everyone. Our experience is that a lot of depression is due to people being afraid of what has happened and what may happen. Alleviating their fear is a great help. We hope that the information in this book and any other you can gather will remove some of your depression.

Pleasure in leisure – the antidote to depression
We believe that isolation can also lead to depression; of course it is equally possible that depression leads to isolation. Meeting volunteer helpers, attending stroke support groups and similar social activities may all help to lessen your depression, both because talking to people who are sympathetic is always encouraging, and sharing worries helps overcome fear of the future.

From our experience one of the most difficult phases of recovery is the time when you are ready to start going out again, meeting friends and enjoying life. You may feel the greatest reluctance to leave your house. This may be for several reasons. Obviously, if you are left seriously disabled, it is physically more difficult to get out. Under these circumstances you may need to adopt a more limited social life, and be prepared to accept help to get about. However, we feel that it is rare for the physical disability actually to be the major restriction; you may, even subconsciously, be using it as an excuse (see Chapter 8).

Perhaps the main reason for reluctance to go out is fear and embarrassment. This is quite understandable. You have probably been ill and even in the hospital for some weeks or months. Then, your friends may be uncertain how to treat you, and some will tell you to 'take it easy'. You may be afraid that you look or sound odd, even mentally abnormal. Some people may treat you as an imbecile. For these and other reasons people recovering from a stroke frequently cut off their social life. This is unnecessary, and one of the worst things that you can do.

Getting out and about   The first step is to wish to meet people. As long as you want to, you will find there are various ways of overcoming your fear. It is probably best to start by inviting people to your own home, where you will feel most relaxed. Once you have overcome your embarrassment, and they theirs, try going to a neighbour's house near by. It is probably best for you to be accompanied by your spouse, or a relative or friend (see also Chapter 8).

Your first visit to a public place may seem the most difficult step to take. After you feel confident about meeting friends in small groups at home or close by in their houses, you need to widen your horizons. It is at this point that therapists or volunteers from a support group can be of the greatest help. They can accompany you to the local shops and stay with you while you buy something. You will soon realize you can manage. In many areas there are clubs organized by the support groups, where you can socialize, play card games or begin drawing and painting. Again, a volunteer can take you there. Sometimes transport is provided free, with any physical assistance you need. Taking part in activities such as this, you will regain your confidence in meeting other people, including strangers.

It is now important that you return to as many of your leisure activities as possible. If you stopped working after the stroke, you may need to develop new hobbies. A lot of hobbies can be continued even by people with considerable physical handicaps. For example, there are facilities for fishing, gardening and bowls for disabled people in our area. Other hobbies are easily taken up, such as most card or board games, stamp collecting or painting. Some people coming to our unit have continued activities such as watch repairing and wood carving, despite having paralysed arms. With determination, and help and advice from others, you should find a range of leisure pursuits that make it worth getting up each morning.

What if I cannot manage at home?

Longterm hospital care is obviously necessary for some people. In our own hospital, only about 5 to 9 per cent of those recovering from a stroke never leave the hospital, either because they cannot be cared for at home or because they have no one at home anyway.

There are, though, non-hospital forms of longterm care. Many people enter nursing homes, where help will be given according to ability while allowing maximum independence. Some of these homes can take married couples. Often trades unions or other friendly societies (the Quakers, for example) run subsidized sheltered housing.

For people who do not stay in the hospital but need constant attention, support for the carers is important. In some hospitals planned hospital admission known as holiday relief is available. This allows the family to have one or two weeks free from nursing. Such schemes rely upon each family taking their relative home after the allotted time, as otherwise future admissions are held up. Access to and information about all these can be obtained from the organizations listed on page 118.

Most people do not have to live away from home or need longterm help from outside organizations once they have regained their confidence. Over 80 per cent of survivors will be in their own homes six months after their stroke, and about 20 per cent of these will probably receive support from some of the services we discussed in Chapter 10. In the next chapter we consider the important question of how the relatives and friends of people living at home after a stroke can be helped.

12 ADJUSTMENT

A stroke can dramatically change the life not only of the sufferer but also of his or her family. Unlike most other disabling diseases, such as arthritis, a stroke happens suddenly, so that there is no time to adapt. Like other acute illnesses such as a heart attack, a stroke is a life-threatening illness. A third factor is that it produces disability that is obvious to all. This combination means that the victim has to adjust both to the acute stress of a serious illness and to any handicap that remains. In this chapter we shall be looking into the psychological reactions experienced by people suffering from stroke and their families, and giving advice on how to cope. The emphasis will be upon what can happen to relationships between people when one of them has had a stroke. We shall also consider the difficulties of caring for someone left moderately or severely disabled, and how these can be eased.

It is often not appreciated how a stroke completely and instantly alters roles within the family. Someone once independent, possibly still at work, is suddenly rendered helpless. The person having a stroke is now a 'patient' who may be incontinent, unable to eat or dress alone, and even be unable to communicate. Not infrequently he or she will be treated as someone of limited intelligence who is talked about in his presence.

The sufferer's reaction

Anyone who has a stroke is immediately thrown into a state of shock – he is unsure of what has happened, afraid of what is going to happen and surprised by the suddenness of events. This state of anxiety and doubt may last anything from a day up to a few weeks. We can call it a stage of crisis.

The second stage is one of treatment. At this time there are high hopes. Most people develop optimistic expectations of recovery, denying that any loss will be permanent. Their feeling is fuelled by the natural rapid recovery that usually occurs over the first few weeks. Optimism is often reinforced because therapy is started. Many people

110

remain in this stage for months, even when it is obvious that recovery will not be complete. Unfortunately, unrealistic therapists and other helpers sometimes build up false hopes of a complete recovery, which ultimately hinder the important adjustment to reality.

At least half of all survivors are left with some handicap, and most will go through a stage of realizing this. For the person who had the stroke, it is one of extreme frustration. He or she is angry with the world. He will compare his present with his previous state of health and become extremely depressed. He can see no worthwhile future. He may give up; a lot of people do not come out of this stage. It is now that counselling from sympathetic, experienced helpers can help, although unfortunately, this is not always available.

The final stage is one of adjustment and acceptance. The disabled person realizes that he or she has to cope with the present state of things. He starts to return to all those activities he can still manage, and develops new interests.

The family's reaction

Not surprisingly, the sudden change in the sufferer's status also causes stress to the family. Once their roles were as spouse or children. Now everyone involved has to take on nursing duties. This is often resented and at first may cause anger directed against the sufferer. Then it is seen to be irrational and can in turn lead to feelings of guilt and depression. If the person with the stroke is in the hospital, the family may feel that they are inadequate and that they should be able to manage at home. Their guilt may expand; they begin to think that they could have prevented the stroke in some way. They also worry about the sufferer when they are not with him.

The first adaptation is to learn to accept your role as carer. For many husbands this is easier than you might expect. As a stroke often occurs around the time of retirement, some easily slip into this new job. Wives, on the other hand, may resent having another 'child' needing care, particularly if they were looking forward to an enjoyable retirement with their husbands. Children may find caring for their parent very difficult. However, we find that most people adapt in the end to their new role of nurse or even parent of the newly dependent person.

The much more difficult adaptation for you all is to allow your relative – often treated as a child – to regain his or her independence. As recovery begins, the once totally dependent person needs to be encouraged to do more. Just as adolescence is often a difficult period, so can the period of recovery be. The carer has to be prepared to reduce the amount of nursing, while the person who had the stroke must become increasingly independent. Both these changes can be hard.

In many ways the reactions you will experience as a family are similar to those after the death of someone in the family. You will probably grieve for the loss of the person you knew. At first your feelings are of extreme anxiety and uncertainty. Each member will be constantly seeking reassurance from everyone else that the sufferer will survive and recover well. Each will note minor differences in the information given: if one doctor says that their relative has a 50 per cent chance of walking again and another that he has a 60 per cent chance, this will be thought to reflect some real improvement. The truth is that neither doctor knew for certain and both gave an approximate answer.

The first days of anxiety are followed by hope as recovery starts. However, even at this stage many relatives start to develop feelings of guilt. They feel responsible for causing the stroke. They blame it upon a minor family quarrel, or upon a job they asked the victim to do, or upon some other imagined cause. These feelings often amount to convictions, but you must accept that in reality you cannot *cause* someone to have a stroke.

As time passes and it becomes obvious that recovery will not be complete, you may all start to develop any number of worries. How will you cope? Will one of you need to stop working to help care for your relative? What about the cost? At the same time, it is common to be angry with the disabled person. He is blamed for his own poor recovery. He is not trying hard enough. Why is he doing this to us? Why should I stop working for her sake?

When someone comes home still needing help, this anger very occasionally turns to physical violence. The strain of caring, coupled with depression, fatigue, frustration and anger can explode. We have seen people who have hit their spouse hard simply out of anger. While physical violence is uncommon, mental cruelty is not unusual. The healthy members of the family simply ignore the dependent person. Yet the continuing anger and frustration only lead to greater feelings of guilt. It is at this stage that professional counselling can be most helpful. If you are suffering from these problems, you should talk to your doctor about them immediately rather than try to hide them.

Help with the psychological stress

These emotions and the changing relationships in your family can lead to considerable psychological stress. This is particularly likely at three crisis points:

1. At the time of the stroke

2. On discharge from the hospital, when people are forced to accept that there may be longterm problems

3. On discharge from any medical or rehabilitative care, forcing the realization that you are now on your own.

The first step is to understand that the feelings we have described are normal. You should feel free to talk about them and encourage others closely involved to discuss their own feelings of anger and guilt. This will help both them and yourself. It is unwise to try and hide your reactions.

You should not hesitate to seek further help with these adjustments. Your doctor will help you come to terms with your feelings and assure you of their normality; other people you can talk to are your minister, psychologists and social workers. Many hospitals run groups for the relatives of stroke patients. These offer a good opportunity to discuss your feelings and share your experiences with other people in the same situation. They also often include educational talks from professional helpers.

It must be faced that sometimes these circumstances cause such stress to already fragile relationships that they bring about separation. Children desert parents. Wives divorce husbands. Some people even feel suicidal. If you feel this is a danger in your case, you must talk to one of the professionals we suggest above.

Personality changes
Some people become quite difficult to live with after a stroke. Major personality changes are rare, but it is not uncommon for previously well controlled characteristics to become more obvious and irritating. The slightly irascible man who used to go outside when angry now becomes a bad-tempered complainer who is always shouting at his family. There is no simple solution. It is probably best to approach the person in the same way one does an awkward child. You should state your limits – 'I'm only giving you a drink once an hour'; you should be consistent, and stick to any conditions you have laid down. You will have to insist that your relative does his fair share. You must be prepared to punish in some way in the last resort – for example, by removing the television. Don't allow yourself to be bullied or to bully.

Look after yourself

Different people react differently to these stresses. Some simply ignore the person with the stroke, expecting others to cope. They continue their own life as before. At the other extreme, some people martyr themselves, devoting every minute of every day to their new-found job. Fortunately, most people who recover from stroke do not need such care, and most people do not react in that way. Nevertheless, anyone faced with caring at home, whether from the start of the stroke or after the person has been in the hospital, needs some guidlines.

Caring for someone who has had a stroke can be hard work. First, there is the physical strain of nursing: lifting, turning, helping to the lavatory. Second, there is the constant worry about whether you are doing enough. Third, there is the difficulty of getting any rest or break. Last, you risk ignoring the rest of your life – your work, friends and family. The key to caring for yourself is:

- Accept help offered
- Seek extra help early
- Ensure you get time off
- Take regular vacations
- Maintain your social life.

You can give proper care only if you are fit and well yourself. Being a martyr does no one any good. It is far better to make your task a pleasant one by allowing yourself regular refreshment than bring physical and mental exhaustion on yourself, and maybe your relative too. Therefore, you must accept any help offered and ask for extra assistance when you need it. Family, friends and neighbours are usually willing to lend a hand if asked. Indeed, many may wish to help but feel that they wil be intruding in some way, or be frightened that their offer may be seen by you as a criticism of your capability. Do not wait until you have failed before you seek help. Instead, make clear immediately what assistance you think you may need.

When accepting help, try to give people jobs they will feel capable of, which they will feel are useful, and which they enjoy. For example, if a neighbour who is a good cook wants to help, ask her to prepare meals for you and the person who has had the stroke. But be careful about asking for nursing help. Ex-nurses and close family will usually be willing, but others may not want to do this sort of job. Remember, too, that your relative may not want acquaintances acting as nurses. There are many other chores that can be taken on by helpers, such as shopping, housework, collecting prescriptions and so on. This will relieve you somewhat and free you for the important work of caring for your relative or spouse.

Getting a break

If the person you are looking after is left with a very severe disability and yet you still want to have him home, you will need to arrange a regular system of relief for yourself. You should have at least one whole day or two half days a week free. You should also try to get two or three weeks' holiday each year.

Freedom during the week can be arranged in various ways. If your family, friends or neighbours are willing and able, you may arrange a schedule that gives you several periods off. Voluntary support groups can often provide relief, either by someone coming to your home or by the dependent person being taken out. Once or twice weekly visits to a hospital stroke unit or a Social Services day centre is another avenue worth exploring. You will probably have to arrange this through your doctor.

During your annual vacation, other members of the family should be able to look after your relative in their home. But you have to be sure that everyone understands the arrangements clearly, and that you are willing to take the dependent person back afterwards. You may not have family who are capable of looking after your relative. You shouldn't feel this excludes you from having a well earned break. Some private and charity-aided nursing homes, homes run by social services and hospitals offer holiday relief. In most countries this help is offered free of charge to those who need it.

Your social life

Someone who is left severely handicapped and totally dependent upon others is unlikely to survive more than a year or two. Less handicapped people still stand a risk of dying in the foreseeable future. You will certainly feel bereft whenever this happens, and it is important that you do not become so engrossed in your caring role that you forget your family and friends. You should continue to invite people to your home and go out to visit them, so maintaining your link with others. This can only benefit your relative too, for the reasons we have already discussed in this chapter.

You should also continue your outside interests. For example, if you used to attend regular weekly or monthly meetings of a club or group, you should try not to miss more than one or two months of them. It is dangerously easy to imagine that you have to give up everything for the sake of the sick person. In the short term (up to eight weeks) this may be so, but it is not in your interest, nor ultimately in the interest of the sick person, to let it go for longer. If you give up all your hobbies and interests you will become depressed very easily and then you will be less efficient in caring for your loved one.

We have written this book from years of firsthand experience with people who have suffered strokes of all kinds and degrees of severity. We have naturally also been in close contact with their families, believing as we do that the best way towards recovery is by the people closest to one another working together to improve every ability that remains. We hope the advice you find here will help you think again when things seem particularly hard, and realize you don't have to, nor should you, face your trouble alone.

FURTHER READING

Caring for the sick authorized by St John Ambulance Association, St Andrew's Ambulance Association and British Red Cross Society, Dorling Kindersley, London, 1983

Chest, Heart and Stroke Association, *Stroke – twenty questions and the answers*
A free leaflet obtainable from the Chest, Heart and Stroke Association, Tavistock House North, Tavistock Square, London WC1H 9JE. Enclose self-addressed stamped envelope.

Darnbrough, A., Kinrade, D., *Directory for disabled people*, 4th ed. (Woodhead-Faulkner, Cambridge, 1985)
A comprehensive guide to practical information and opportunities for disabled and handicapped people. Includes useful addresses.

Isaacs, B., *Understanding stroke* (Chest, Heart and Stroke Association, London 1985)
A 32 page booklet.

Hale, G., *The new source book for the disabled* (Heinemann, London 1983)
An illustrated guide to easier and more independent living for physically disabled people, their families and friends. Includes 'resources' section.

Hewson, L., *When half is whole* (Dove Communications, Blackburn, Australia)
A well written book describing the effects of stroke; written by an occupational therapist who has herself suffered a stroke and recovered.

Law, D., Paterson, B., *Living after a stroke* (Souvenir Press, London 1980)
Biography of Diana Law and her recovery from stroke.

Mental Health Foundation, *Someone to talk to directory* (Routledge & Kegan Paul, London 1985)
A directory of self-help and community support agencies – national and local – in the United Kingdom and Republic of Ireland.

Mobility Information Service, *Driving after a stroke* (Mobility Information Service, Copthorne Community Hall, Shelton Road, Shrewsbury, Shropshire SY3 8TD, Shrewsbury 1984)

Moss Rehabilitation Hospital, *In the driver's seat – some questions and answers about driver training for the stroke patient*
A free pamphlet from the Moss Rehabilitation Hospital, Box LL, 12th St. and Tabor Road, Philadelphia PA 19141, USA; enclose self-addressed stamped envelope.

Rose, F.C., Capildeo, R., *Stroke: the facts*. (Oxford University Press, Oxford, 1981).

Sahs, A.L., Hartman, E.C., Aronson, S.M., *Guidelines for Stroke Care* (US Department of Health, Education and Welfare Publication No (HRA) 76–14017). Lists agencies and services including National Easter Seal Society for Crippled Children and Adults, Visiting Nurse Association, Mental Health Association, Home Health Agencies, American Heart Association, Local Health Department Home Health Agency, Family Service Agency, Meals-on-wheels, Homemaker-home Health Aide Agency, Community Mental Health Center, Hospital Social Work Program, American Red Cross, Salvation Army, Public Health Nurse, Vocational Rehabilitation Service, Arthritis Foundation

Wade, D.T., Langton Hewer R., Skilbeck, C.E., David, R.M., *Stroke: a critical approach to diagnosis, treatment and management* (Chapman Hall, London, 1985)
Gives the evidence underlying the statements made in this book.

USEFUL ADDRESSES

UNITED KINGDOM

Association of Crossroads Care Attendant Schemes Ltd
94 Coton Road
Rugby
Warwickshire CV21 4LN

The British Red Cross Society
9 Grosvenor Crescent
London SW1X 7EJ

Chest, Heart and Stroke Association
Tavistock House North
Tavistock Square
London WC1H 9JE

Chest, Heart and Stroke Association Scottish Branch
65 North Castle Street
Edinburgh EH2 3LT

The Northern Ireland Chest, Heart and Stroke Association
21 Dublin Road
Belfast BT2 7FJ

The Disabled Living Foundation
380–384 Harrow Road
London W9 2HU

The Royal Association for Disability and Rehabilitation (RADAR)
25 Mortimer Street
London W1N 8AB

UNITED STATES

American Red Cross
National Headquarters
17th and D Streets
Washington, DC 20006

International Center for the Disabled
340 East 24th Street
New York, NY 10010

Sister Kenny Institute
800 East 28th Street at Chicago Avenue
Minneapolis, MN 55407

Stroke Club International
805 12th Street
Galveston, TX 77550

Stroke Foundation
898 Park Avenue
New York, NY 10021

CANADA

Canadian Association of Social Workers
55 Parkdale Avenue
4th Floor
Ottawa, Ontario
K1Y 1E5

Canadian Medical Association
1867 Alta Vista Drive
Ottawa, Ontario
K1N 7B7

Care Professionals
253 Danforth Avenue
Suite 200
Toronto, Ontario
M4K 1N2

Heart and Stroke Foundation
576 Church Street
Toronto, Ontario
M4Y 2S1

Manitoba Stroke Club Inc
213–93 Lombard Avenue
Winnipeg, Manitoba
R3B 3B1

Quebec Stroke Recovery
  Association
135 Sherbrooke Street East
Suite 1002
Montreal, Quebec
H2Y 1G6

Secretariat for Fitness in Third
  Age
c/o CP/RA
333 River Road
Ottawa, Ontario
K1L 8H9

Stroke Association of B.C.
1645 West 10th Avenue
Vancouver, British Columbia
V6J 2A2

Stroke Recovery Association
c/o Jenny Halverson, OT
Queen Elizabeth Hospital
Box 660
Charlottetown, Prince Edward
  Island
C1A 8T5

Stroke Recovery Association
170 Donway West
Don Mills, Ontario
M3C 2G3

Stroke Recovery Association
c/o Department of Occupational
  Therapy

The University of Alberta
Edmonton, Alberta
T6G 2G4

Stroke Recovery Association
c/o Prof Valerie Gilbey
265 Massey Street
Fredrickton, New Brunswick
E3B 2Z5

Stroke Recovery Association
c/o Roma Aiken
2 Avon Crescent
Halifax, Nova Scotia
B3R 2E3

Stroke Recovery Association
c/o Ian Gulliver
21 Smith Avenue
St John's, Newfoundland
A1C 5E8

Stroke Recovery Association
122 Assiniboine Drive
Saskatoon, Saskatchewan
S7K 1H7

Victoria Order of Nurses
500 Cummer Avenue
Willowdale, Ontario
M2M 2G5

AUSTRALIA

Mrs Frank Brewer
Speech Pathologist
Douglas Parker Rehabilitation
  Centre
31 Tower Road
Newtown
Tasmania 7008

Ms Cecily Cox
Support Self-Help & Social
  Activities for Stroke People

PO Box 126
Manly
Queensland 4179

Pauline Farrestall
Secretary
The Adelaide Stroke Club
33 Gawan Road
Para Hills South Australia 5096

Ms Clare Grey
Brass Stroke Support Group
PO Box 226
Geelong
Victoria 3220

Ms Mardie O'Sullivan
President
The Stroke Association of
  Western Australia
PO Box 265
Nedlands
Western Australia 6009

Anita Rosenberg
President
The Straight Talk and Stroke
  Club
1 Bedford Street
Surry Hills
NSW 2010

Gordon and Eve Williamson
132 Kunyuny Road
Mt Eliza
Victoria 3930

Helen Vadas
Speech Pathologist
Caulfield Hospital
294 Kooyong Road
Caulfield
Victoria 3162

ACKNOWLEDGMENTS

Our first acknowledgment must be to all our patients, their families and friends; without their probing questions we could give no answers. Second, we are grateful to all those who have worked in the Frenchay Stroke Unit, past and present. Many of their constant and constructive comments are reflected in the ideas we have expressed here. Third, we are grateful to the Department of Health and Social Security, the Bristol Council for Voluntary Services, the Chest Heart and Stroke Association and all the other organizations that have supported the Unit financially and allowed us to conduct our research, much of which forms the basis for this book. Fourth, we acknowledge Dr Pamela Enderby's help and advice with Chapter 9, and Mrs Meg Holbrook, on whose study of the reactions of victims and families of stroke we were able to draw. Last, we are grateful for the patience of our own families while we have been writing this book.

RLH

DTW

The publishers would like to thank the following for their help in the preparation of this book:
For permission to reproduce the photographs: Chest, Heart and Stroke Association Scottish Branch, Edinburgh (page 78; photograph courtesy of *Glasgow South and Eastwood Extra*); Frenchay Hospital, Bristol (page 46); NOMEQ, NI Medical, Redditch, Worcestershire (page 66); Picker International Ltd, Wembley, Middlesex (page 45); Searle Pharmaceuticals, High Wycombe, Buckinghamshire and Dr G Beevers, Consultant Physician, Dudley Road Hospital, Birmingham (page 22).
We would also like to thank Nottingham Rehab, West Bridgford, Nottingham for permission to reproduce photographs (page 99, *below*, 100, *left*) and for lending equipment for photographs (page 99, *above*, 102).
The photographs on pages 52, 68, 70, 71, 73, 74, 77, 99, *above*, 100, *right* and 102 were taken by Ray Moller, assisted by Liz Gedney. The modelling was by Anne and David Jones, and Esther Hingle. Props were kindly lent by Dorma, Swinton, Manchester and The Reject Shop, London W1.
We thank Mrs Lesley Bradley, MCSP, Physiotherapist at the Stroke Unit, Frenchay Hospital, Bristol for her advice and supervision of the exercise sequences and care photographs.
The diagrams are by Kevin Marks.

INDEX

Page numbers in *italic* refer to the illustrations